Horses and Human Health

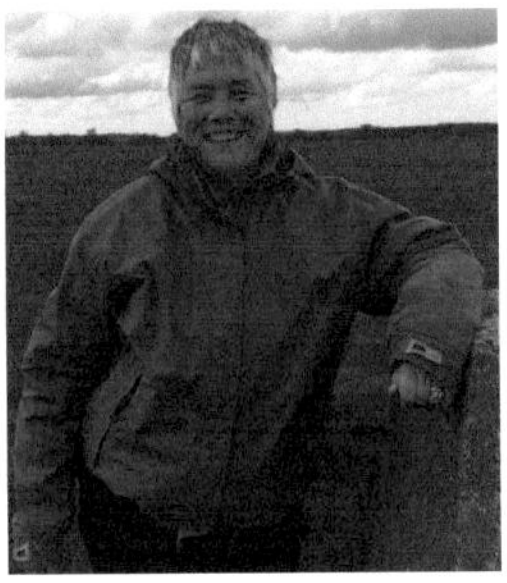

I have been using horses to improve human health for more than thirty years. I first became aware of the therapeutic impact and importance of involving horses whilst helping others back to health in the 1980s.

Since that time I have gained a considerable understanding of the field and in 2003 developed an Outdoor Therapy Centre in Wiltshire alongside my mainstream work in NHS General Practice.

As a doctor I know that medicine doesn't hold all the answers and am pleased to use the full range of outdoor therapy in my practice. I have taught many, lectured widely and now recognise the need to establish a book to support the development of these therapies into the UK. My dream is that outdoor therapy, and horse based therapy in particular, is more available to people as the understanding of this work is spread.

A block to the wider usage of horses in the field of human health is its complexity. To overcome this I have developed the matrix approach which I now use in practice. I hope you will also find this useful, both in practice and in the explanation of this work. I also hope you will be encouraged to explore and expand this important and rewarding field further.

I wish to thank all who helped to produce this book. A book is never the work of only one person.

Horses and Human Health

Dr Celia Grummitt

First published in 2016 by GUL

British Library Cataloguing-in-Publication data
A catalogue record for this book is available from the British Library

Typeset and printed by Riverside Publishing Solutions Ltd, Lower Woodford, Salisbury, Wiltshire, UK

Contents

1 Setting the scene **1**

1.0 Horses and human health 1

1.1 Widening the availability 3

1.2 Matrices 4

1.3 Definitions 7

2 Outdoor therapy **17**

2.0 The importance of environment 17

2.1 Being outside 18

2.2 Outside and engaged 19

2.3 Biophilia 19

2.4 Outdoor therapy and its history 21

3 Horses, the extra factor **25**

3.0 Why horses? 25

3.1 The physical effects 25

3.2 Horses and emotions 26

3.3 Horses and reflection 27

3.4 Horse character and personality 28

3.5 Horses in therapeutic intervention 29

3.6 Choice of horse 33

4 The matrix expanded **37**

4.0 Areas of application 37

4.1 Therapeutic interventions 38

4.2 Levels of therapy 39

4.3 Considerations in therapy 40

4.4 The horse based therapy matrix 44

4.5 Therapeutic interventions expanded and explained 44

4.6 Horse based areas of application 57

4.7 Endless possibilities 67

5 Selection, training and care of horses for therapy **73**
5.0 Selection of therapy horses 73
5.1 Characteristics of therapy horses 74
5.2 Training for therapy 75
5.3 The care of the therapy horse 78

6 Measuring for success **81**
6.0 The purpose of recording and measuring 81
6.1 How to measure success 82
6.2 Analysis 92
6.3 Why measure? 92

7 Moving on to practise safely **95**
7.0 The team 95
7.1 The self 98
7.2 Matrix and boundaries 101
7.3 The emergency dismount 102
7.4 The organisational umbrella 108
7.5 The "perfect pathway" 114
7.6 In summary 119

Chapter 1

Setting the scene

1.0 Horses and human health

My intention in writing this book is to give people an understanding of how horses affect human health in a positive way and what horses can offer when used therapeutically.

"The horse is an interactive being and brings an entire new dimension to the therapeutic intervention".

This book is designed to provide the glue between a variety of human focussed skills and sound equine knowledge, so that they can be used together effectively, professionally and safely. The glue is essential if the two areas are to be used in a complementary and symbiotic manner. This is how horses are used to assist humans.

One of the challenges to nationwide recognition of the use of horses in this way is the complexity which is greater than many realise. Those starting to work in this area usually do not realise its full potential. Emerging schools of practice, often heralded by their founders as the only way, are actually only part of the whole picture. They are one way of delivering the benefits and outcomes sought for the recipient but, just as many computer programmes allow the user to choose a path to reach an outcome that works logically for them, there will be other ways to achieve the same.

If the psychological aspect interests either the practitioner or the recipient more than other areas, they will choose an intervention that includes this language. The same is true of those preferring the physical elements or educational aspects of the therapeutic intervention.

I will show how either can be seen as correct but cannot happen in isolation, as more than one area of a person's life will be affected by this work, whether that was the intended outcome or not.

This book is careful not to exclude any practice by use of reserved language or unnecessary requirements. It also seeks to define effective, professional and safe practice to inform all interested parties, whether providers, participants or purchasers. The territorial practice of "naming and claiming" that can occur in emerging fields of innovative practice only causes confusion and compounds the lack of credibility for the therapeutic area as a whole.

The outdoor environment adds improved concentration, improved mood, greater motivation and enhanced sense of perception.

The realisation of the increased effectiveness of using therapeutic interventions out of doors is finally becoming more widely accepted in the United Kingdom. Until recently, physical and mental health therapies have been practised mainly inside buildings. The importance of the style of the indoor environment in improving outcomes is now better understood and therefore changing. There is also an increasing understanding of the positive effect that the outdoor environment provides and some therapists are taking their sessions outside.

They are starting to walk with people rather than sit at a conventional desk. Therapists now may engage in gardening, climbing and working in a wilderness to name but a few applications. This movement is gaining strength and this brings opportunity to mainstream a very powerful therapeutic area.

All practitioners should be considering whether to take their work outside whenever appropriate. Similarly, students of health, education, equine work, psychology, health sciences and outdoor pursuits should be being encouraged to understand how the environment in which they work affects the outcomes in their field.

The general benefits of exercise are well understood and described but whilst gym based activity will have a good effect physically, exercise taken outside has a wider therapeutic effect. The outdoor environment adds improved concentration, improved mood, greater motivation and an enhanced sense of perception. This is discussed in more depth in the next chapter. Horses will be shown to provide yet more benefit to certain therapeutic interventions and are an asset the country cannot afford to ignore in it's search for more effective health and wellbeing solutions without greater cost.

Horses affect human health positively on various levels but for a few individuals they can also affect health in a negative way through allergy or injury. Horses are large, powerful, fright or flight, prey animals and interaction with them is not without risk. This may perhaps add to their potential for some people.

Whilst outdoor therapy can take place in most settings, horse based work cannot. The effort required to access it is outweighed by the advantages it provides but this isn't yet widely understood. A therapist, two bicycles and a person engaged in therapy will produce useful work at many levels. The replacement of the bicycles with a horse provides a vastly increased array of opportunities for the therapist to use and this may at first seem bewildering. The horse is an interactive being and brings an entire a whole new dimension to the therapeutic intervention.

1.1 Widening the availability

There is an opportunity to widen the availability of horse based therapy country wide by simply enabling horses of mainstream riding centres to be used.

Many riding schools are already aware of how horses affect human health in a positive way and may be involved in a level of therapeutic intervention without calling it by that name. Some may never have considered a role within therapeutic provision, whilst others may

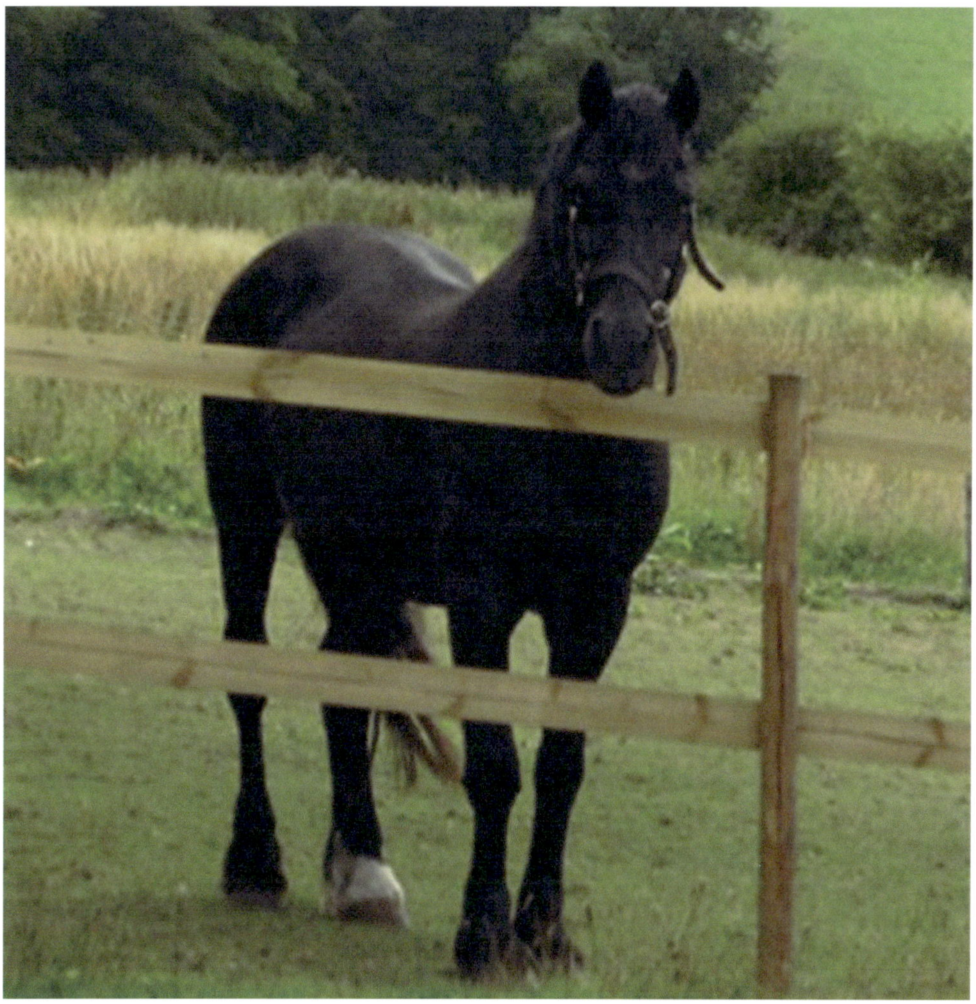

Image 1: Caemansel Prince who helped me begin horse based therapy

have considered specialist groups already working from their premises to be the experts rather than themselves.

If it were possible to include more mainstream riding centres in this area of work then my aim in writing this book would have been realised.

The complexity of the field of "horses and human health" has been referred to already, as well as the fact that therapy for the improvement of wellbeing can be very simple. The level of therapy offered by a centre needs to be one that all are comfortable with and in which all are confident. The reasonable fear of accidental involvement in a session that is too challenging can be managed by a clear statement of what can be offered at the outset. Even an apparently simple provision of opportunities for volunteering needs to be clearly outlined as not all volunteers are equally able.

As in all areas, strength, resilience and capability for this therapeutic intervention comes from teamworking and this is covered in more depth later.

It is hoped that the reader is now beginning to see the scope of horse based therapy and the potential for offering or accessing therapy at a level which suits their situation. Hopefully providers have also seen that they could be involved in this work, offering services that are effective, professional and safe to certain groups of people in need, once they are in possession of appropriate understanding.

1.2 Matrices

When an area of work is complex and hard to grasp it is best to try and simplify it. A useful exercise is to capture all the information on one side of A4 paper. Any attempts to widen the subject or to go into more detail are to be strongly resisted. What follows is a distillation of knowledge gained through years of working in many and varied settings – the use of the matrix.

A matrix is a mathematical tool designed to enable the possibility of interconnection between multiple factors to be understood. An example matrix is shown. (Fig. 1.)

The matrix is in the expected mathematical format and the x and y axes have typical numerical or algebraic values.

In the completed squares just 4 examples are given of how the square could be named or, put another way, what factors would operate within the square.

These are 4 out of the 35 possible options or combinations shown on this matrix.

Fig. 2 shows a more complex matrix which is suited to therapy work. In it, the values of the x and y axes are expanded as they might not have numerical values but may be written

Fig. 1: Example of a mathematical matrix

	A	B	C	D	E
1					
2		2b			
3					
4					4e
5				5d	
6		6b			
7					

concepts or applications. In the matrix below (Fig. 2) the boxes marked by "x" show possible connections in a similar way and again mark 5 out of 96 possibilities.

The upper left area is used for noting any overarching rules or external factors which may have an effect on either, or both, sets of parameters.

Fig. 2: An example matrix

	A set of parameters												
Overarching rules or considerations													
A set of parameters													
				X									
				X									
						X							
		X		X									

This is explained further in the coloured matrix in Fig. 3 and the first steps are taken to applying the use of the matrix to the field of outdoor therapy as a whole.

Each zone of the matrix below has a different shade of background colour for ease of reference.

There is no green so lets say the first box, top left, entitled Level, refers to the level of complexity at which the offer of therapy can be provided. This is defined by, or defines, the level of experience and capacity of the team.

The darkest area, that of areas of application, are the activities offered in which therapeutic intervention can take place.

The therapeutic interventions offered are shown in the large box on the left hand side leaving the main part of the matrix, the palest area, to show the possible connections between activity and therapy.

The considerations shown on the top between Level an Areas of application are the overarching rules or external factors which apply in respect to this matrix, for example, limited car parking, no disabled access, poor weather conditions and so on.

Now that a basic understanding of the type of matrix used is set out it can be developed into the working model.

Fig. 3: Coloured matrix

<table>
<tr><td>Level</td><td>Considerations</td><td colspan="10">Areas of application</td></tr>
<tr><td></td><td></td><td></td><td></td><td></td><td></td><td></td><td></td><td></td><td></td><td></td><td></td></tr>
<tr><td colspan="2">Therapeutic interventions offered</td><td colspan="10">Possibilities</td></tr>
<tr><td colspan="2"></td><td></td><td></td><td></td><td></td><td></td><td></td><td></td><td></td><td></td><td></td></tr>
<tr><td colspan="2"></td><td></td><td></td><td></td><td></td><td></td><td></td><td></td><td></td><td></td><td></td></tr>
<tr><td colspan="2"></td><td></td><td></td><td></td><td></td><td></td><td></td><td></td><td></td><td></td><td></td></tr>
<tr><td colspan="2"></td><td></td><td></td><td></td><td></td><td></td><td></td><td></td><td></td><td></td><td></td></tr>
<tr><td colspan="2"></td><td></td><td></td><td></td><td></td><td></td><td></td><td></td><td></td><td></td><td></td></tr>
<tr><td colspan="2"></td><td></td><td></td><td></td><td></td><td></td><td></td><td></td><td></td><td></td><td></td></tr>
</table>

1.3 Definitions

When working in any subject area definitions are helpful. As has already been alluded to, there are an alarming array of titles, words, techniques and languages in use in this growing work. The terms and phrases used to describe it have changed in the last few years and will continue to do so. This book will focus on basic definitions which are sufficient to describe work in this field but will aim to stay away from current "in vogue" terminology.

1.3.1 Horse

In some areas of the work the term "equine" is used more than horse as it includes both horses and ponies. Both terms are equally valuable in the work. People with horse knowledge know the difference between horses and ponies to be based on size alone with the horse being 14.2 hands or above and a pony being below 14.2 hands. The term "horse" is used throughout this book to denote an equine of any height, gender, personality, breed or age. This is to enable commissioners, funders of the therapy or indeed potential beneficiaries, to understand and feel comfortable with the terminology.

The international organisation HETI (Horses in Education and Therapy International), uses the word "horse" for the same reason as most non-riders identify all equines by this term.

1.3.2 Therapy

A medical definition of therapy is an intervention designed to improve either the physical, mental or emotional well-being of an individual. At its simplest a therapeutic intervention

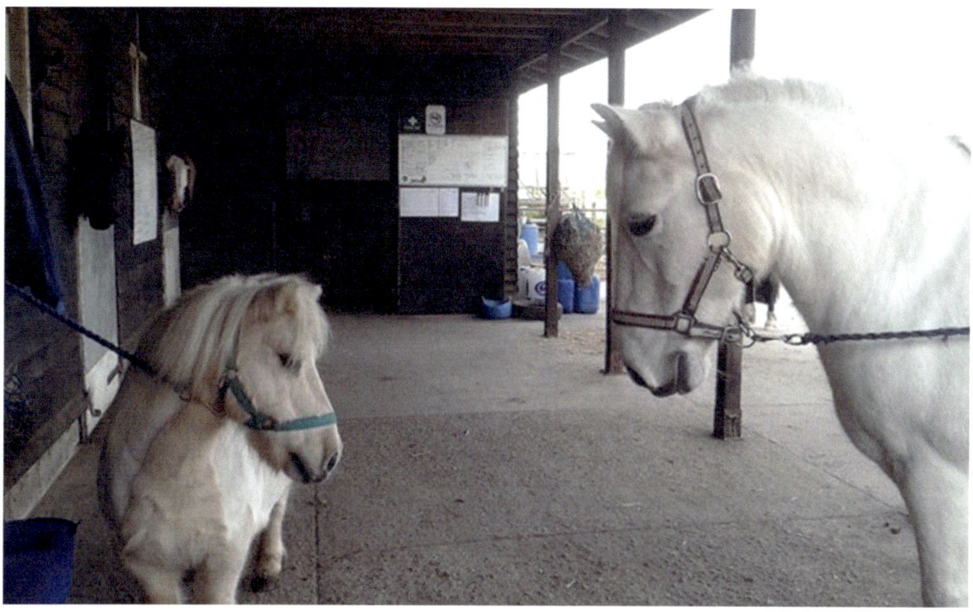

Image 2: Little and Large

could be a smile exchanged with a passer-by, a cake baked and delivered to a new neighbour, or time spent outside with an empathetic individual and a horse.

At the other end of the scale a therapeutic intervention could be a challenging and professionally led activity designed to move someone physically, mentally or emotionally from a currently held position or belief towards a new and healthier state. All the above will have a positive effect on the mood of the recipient and may cover widely varying outcomes such as:-

- Reduced stress with potential reduction in blood pressure and lower cardiac risk
- Reduced back pain
- Happier family members
- Hope of future life leading to more active social engagements
- Increased joint mobility
- Reduction in post traumatic stress disorder symptoms
- Enhanced sense of self esteem or achievement

1.3.3 Therapist

A therapist is someone with a recognisable qualification in improving human physical, mental or emotional health or human behaviour. A secondary outcome of any improvement in the above will be an improvement in the well-being of the recipient. A therapist's qualification should be recognised at national level and allow them to work in autonomous practice in their field with an understanding of their own limitations, the need for supervision and when to refer on as appropriate.

A therapy assistant is someone with basic knowledge in the field of improving human physical, mental or emotional health or human behaviour but who doesn't hold a qualification sufficient to allow independent practice. In the health, education, equine or outdoor pursuits fields this is easily understood as all workers move up through similar systems for example level 1 coaches holding the CIEC (certificate in equestrian coaching) have a relevant qualification to work under the supervision of a level 2 coach in a similar way to a rehabilitation assistant working under the supervision of a physiotherapist or a newly qualified counsellor.

The field of horse based therapy is no different. If this field of therapy is to be taken seriously, those working within it will need to be able to describe their competencies in such a way that the outside world can understand and relate to. A riding coach is clearly skilled in the area of improving riding, and will have coaching skills, but may not be suited to working in the field of horse based therapy.

Fig. 4: Bell curve showing a normal distribution

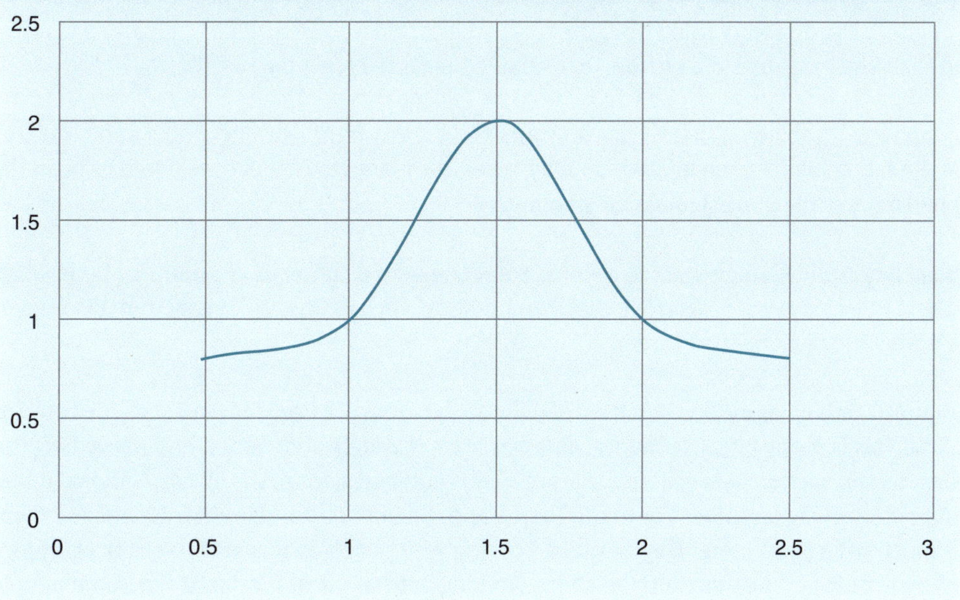

1.3.4 Normality

It is important to note that normal does not mean perfect (no one is perfect, though some may believe they are). Normal means "good enough" or being within the central range of a bell curve distribution of a population, see Fig. 4.

Being within the normal range for the height at any age, or for intelligence, is a better way of referring to a "normal" state.

All riding coaches know, and regularly see, how variations in body shape and flexibility of "normal people" can adversely affect how a horse goes for them under saddle. This is where the opportunity arises for the riding coach to further their work. This could be termed a therapeutic intervention if the improvement leads to benefits beyond that expected, perhaps by also improving the self esteem or confidence of an anxious person.

1.3.5 Rehabilitation

The World Health Organisation's definition of rehabilitation is used nationally within the UK and firmly places the act of rehabilitation within the therapeutic range of provision. It states that rehabilitation is an active process by which those disabled by injury or disease achieve a full recovery or, if that is not possible, realise their optimal physical, mental and social potential and are integrated into their most appropriate environment.

1.3.6 Disability and disadvantage

The term disabled tends to be applied to those with a specific physical or mental lack of function. The disability could be caused by genetics, birth trauma, illness or injury and refers to that which disables the person, for example their loss of hearing or epilepsy.

A learning disability is one which prevents the person from learning at the same rate, or assimilating information in a similar way, when compared to others considered to be in the main body of the normal range for learning.

Disability could also be used to refer to someone with disordered emotions or behaviours where these have arisen from a long term condition, such as an autistic spectrum disorder or a borderline personality disorder.

Mental illness or injury is as much a disability as the a loss of a limb but isn't always treated as such. This is partly because mental illnesses are not widely understood and partly because they can be overlooked as there are less obvious outward signs of the illness. National initiatives are seeking to address both the stigma and the under resourcing in this field and there is much work to be done. The therapist working with people in this area needs to be appropriately qualified just as much as those working with physical disability. For some people with complex needs the therapy is best delivered by a team approach to ensure all areas of need can be therapeutically covered.

A disability of any kind may be temporary and improve in response to a rehabilitation programme, or it could be permanent where no further improvement is expected.

Disadvantage is an increasingly used term and covers all disabilities but includes the wider, unfavourable conditions which may affect a person's ability to live within the normal range. It covers environmental factors such as poor parenting, poverty, and social exclusion. It may be used as a reason for abnormal but as yet unattributed behaviour which has arisen from a lack of understanding or acceptance of society's norms. Disadvantage is becoming an umbrella term for all who would benefit from therapeutic interventions and is a clear example of how definitions change within this field.

1.3.7 Emotions

No book about therapy would be complete without a working understanding of emotion. Emotions affect every human on the planet, encompassing both their own emotions and those of other people. An emotion is a feeling and often described as something intuitive rather than cognitive, i.e. felt not thought. A person's personality and life experiences will affect how much the emotions are displayed or even acknowledged, but all have them. One of the functions of our emotions is to help make sense of the world and therefore an imbalance or disorder in emotion will lead to adverse health consequences if left unaddressed.

Feelings such as happiness, sadness, guilt, fear, confusion and hope are aroused by events which may be linked to words or senses such as touch or sight. Emotions are said to add colour to life as they deepen the response felt to a trigger, whether positively or negatively. They assist with relationships and are so visceral that they can cause physical symptoms, usually to help with the fight or flight response.

Emotions arise in the brain and are thought to originate from the limbic system which is situated between the brain stem and the cortex. The brain stem provides core functions of living such as breathing without the need for thought and the cortex is where reasoning and thinking take place.

Mankind has had emotions from the start and they are thought to have been a main communication method for cave dwelling man. Literature recognised emotion rather than passion many centuries ago and those who would like to suggest they are a new and perhaps unnecessary invention would be misguided.

All humans experience emotional responses to daily events which are then processed by the brain. An understanding of emotion is therefore needed in the therapeutic setting because emotional responses will not only be triggered in the recipient and the therapist, but also in any horse involved.

1.3.8 Empathy versus sympathy

No list of definitions in a guide about therapeutic interventions would be complete without the inclusion of empathy and sympathy. This is because in such a setting, with horses or without, a therapy team should be using empathy rather than sympathy. In sympathy the ability is to share the person's emotions and respond with care and or pity. In empathy it is the ability to understand and identify with a person in their situation but not produce a personal response to it. This both enhances any therapeutic input and protects the therapists from emotional overload.

1.3.9 Handing back and referring on

In all therapeutic areas, whichever aspect of health, education or wellbeing is involved, there needs to be an understanding of the following:-

- handing back care
- referring on
- the lead therapist role

This is used in practice across many professions and happens frequently in the horse world. A horse may go away for foaling or schooling and later be handed back to the owner. A horse may be too good or too ambitious for a riding centre and be referred on to a private competition home. A yard manager might set out a plan of poulticing for a particular horse, which the groom follows, and the yard manager reviews. This is about working to strengths and being aware of areas of weakness.

Handing back and referring on ensures the correct passing of responsibility to another when a therapeutic intervention is closed.

A lead therapist is the one holding the responsibility of the intervention or programme even if an assistant or another therapist is involved in the delivery of the treatment package.

Case study 1

Jeff was referred to Gul (a Level 3 Outdoor Therapy Centre) by his Primary School Teacher. The School had used therapeutic activities at Gul before for young people who were struggling in class. Jeff's referral letter stated he struggled with his class size, concentration, manual dexterity and all forms of social interaction. School hinted, most professionally, that the home circumstances were not calm. Jeff lived with his mother who had a new partner and several ex partners, one of whom was Jeff's father. It appeared that Jeff was sometimes used to create difficulties between his mother and father. Jeff was an only child.

As a result of his mother's slightly chaotic lifestyle Jeff had experienced 4 house moves and 3 schools in his first 8 years of life. Jeff was now 9.

Jeff was not subject to a formal Statement of Special Educational Need but was being helped by a teaching assistant giving him one-to-one attention for part of the school day. The school reported that Jeff was behind in reading, writing and maths. However, when matters were discussed verbally or children were asked to report back after listening to a story, he was able to perform in line with other members of the class and his age group.

Jeff and his mother came together for the assessment. Mother did not drive so his step father brought them. It was noted that his mother was not comfortable with the outdoor environment and was certainly not dressed for it. Jeff wasn't dressed for it either so the team used the stores of spare clothing and footwear held on site to dress him more appropriately for his time at the yard. Mother confessed to her fear of horses. Jeff was assessed by a senior therapist and the horse chosen for the assessment was an aged, calm, aloof Highland called MacDuff. When Jeff arrived, MacDuff was tied up and standing quietly in the yard, munching contentedly from a hay net.

Jeff was observed with his mother and their interactions noted, including his need for attention and his permanent state of agitation Jeff happily went with the assessing therapist into the yard, whilst his mother remained on the other side of the fence.

Jeff was not frightened of horses, he was fascinated. He was keen to move around so he was encouraged to run around the small triangle of grass directly outside the yard to "warm up". Much of this was done being an aeroplane. Jeff did not display any particular clumsiness, abnormal gait or laziness. When the therapist felt the time was right, Jeff was asked to come into the yard to be introduced to MacDuff. He was told in a calm voice that horses didn't like people shouting, flapping or running too close to them and that he would need to remember this. It was noticed that Jeff followed these instructions well. The instructions given were short and concise but these caused him no problem and he was compliant. He was good with the grooming, surprisingly so, and much of his agitation settled during that interaction.

In this new environment, Jeff did not question boundaries nor try to push them. As he had one-to-one attention, he had no need to seek for more. In addition it was noticed that he liked the feel of the horse and also lent forward to smell the horse. Jeff was chatty throughout the interaction, in fact he rarely stopped talking.

Whilst Jeff was in the yard having his assessment his mother was enjoying her chat with the Yard Mummy of the day. This Level 3 Centre is a charity where the specific role of Yard Mummy fulfils the role of meeting and greeting everyone, with time to listen to relatives, friends and beneficiaries alike.

Their chat covered many things including looking after Jeff at home and how he could be difficult to settle at bedtime, how his behaviour worsened when weekends with his father were expected. His mother's anger about this situation was quite apparent. The Yard Mummy felt that the speech content suggested Jeff was seen as a nuisance by his mother, slightly more than is normal for most 9 year old children. This might have been due to his mother's wish to concentrate on her new relationship.

The assessing therapist asked Jeff if he would like to sit on the horse. This is often done at an assessment to see whether anxiety is a major factor or is easily overcome. Jeff was keen to sit on MacDuff so was explained to him that he would need to wear a riding hat. Jeff made it successfully back to the office, had a riding hat fitted and told his mother he was going to go riding now. Her reaction was interesting. She was anxious about this and the therapy Team gently informed her that all would be well and that her fears shouldn't be allowed to affect Jeff's session.

A side walker was arranged, the horse made ready with a back pad and bridle. Jeff was asked to wait on the top of the yards' wide mounting block. He did this very well and with very little agitation. His attention was focussed on the horse being brought round. He followed advice and mounted well and confidently. He said he would like the therapist to hold his leg when that was offered. Apart from an exclamation when the horse started to move off in walk, Jeff rode with a smile throughout.

He enjoyed feeling the movement. It was noticed that his core stability and body awareness were adequate to ride safely. He was able to reposition his body in accordance with suggestions from the therapist who was also a riding coach. He enjoyed reaching forward and playing with the wither end of the mane. Jeff was able to look up at the trees in the distance and count the birds. He asked to repeat the small walk when the first circuit had been completed. Jeff was asked if he would like to come again and he was very clear that he would like this very much.

At the end of the assessment, another member of staff engaged Jeff with some horse related activities which enabled the assessing therapist, yard mummy and Jeff's mother to have a quick discussion. The Recovery Star was shown and explained, but not completed because this does not happen until the first session. The Outdoor Therapy, Horse Therapy and Education Matrices were also shown to his mother.

The therapist advised that Gul would be in touch with his school to confirm what was being arranged or offered. It was felt that Jeff would begin with a few weeks of one-to-one sessions to ensure he was safe and confident at the yard. Then he could move into sessions with others to help with the learning of social interaction skills. The therapist asked whether any consideration had been given for a more formal medical assessment of Jeff's difficulties and his mother replied it had not.

Whilst Jeff certainly displayed some behaviours that would indicate attention deficit issues these were not extreme and could alternatively have been explained by difficulty with attachment and his experiences of parenting. This was clearly not discussed with mother.

It was decided that Jeff would benefit from:-

1. Physical activity – time outside getting dirty
2. Being enabled to succeed
3. Learning to communicate
4. Educational input

It was not felt that Jeff needed any form of physical therapy and that his psychological wellbeing would be observed and feedback given. The matrix was completed in accordance with this and with the expectation that he would start a horse based programme. The horse had successfully calmed him, aided concentration, carried him and delighted him, all of which would serve well in helping him to develop certain skills.

After feedback to the school, it was agreed that Jeff would attend for two mornings a week for an hour and a half session each time. It was also agreed that his grandparents would fund a further hour in an after school slot on another day, to be part of the Stable Club programme when he was considered ready.

Mother had clearly enjoyed their visit to Gul and had been listened to, but equally was somewhat bemused by the whole process and especially that Jeff found it as pleasing as he did.

The Recovery Star goals were was set as:-

1. Learning a new skill in riding a horse
2. Learning to look after a horse through horse care
3. Learning to be calm and useful on the yard as part of the team
4. Learning to communicate better with others described to Jeff as "Learning to listen and to speak well"
5. Learning to understand and be understood

It was agreed that horse agility would be a good tool to use for this.

Conclusion

After six weeks on the programme, Jeff was reviewed. School had already seen a change in his behaviour with better concentration in lessons. Mother had come to terms with the fact that some boys liked to be dirty and be outside, this wasn't simply Jeff displaying characteristics of the ex-partner whom she disliked. Jeff then joined Cubs and achieved outdoor activities in that way, he also joined the School Football Team and proved to be a good player. School reduced Jeff 's sessions to one a week but his grandparents continued the Stable Club. After a further term, Jeff stopped attending during the school day and returned to mainstream education whilst continuing his Stable Club attendance. In school holidays Jeff would attend for Bushcraft activities which he equally enjoyed.

Chapter 2
Outdoor therapy

2.0 The importance of environment

Environment matters and this is increasingly understood. A poor environment will exert a detrimental effect on a person or group of people. A good one will exert a positive effect. So strongly does environment affect people that it is used to alter human behaviour on a daily basis.

In every day walks of life colours, noise, internal decoration, smells and the use of space, both inside and out, are used to create specific responses in people. This is useful not least because the response elicited is reproducible in most people exposed to that particular environment, even if there will always be exceptions to this rule.

The study of the environment for better health care provision, to promote the sale of goods, to increase productivity in offices and ensure smoother movement of people through shopping precincts keeps entire industries in work on a daily basis.

The use of environment enhancing devices such as air fresheners, scented candles and soft furnishings are all attempts to change or improve the environment.

Environment is used to change or affect human behaviour and so it is not surprising that environment has a large part to play in therapy. The environment in health care, in sales, in office spaces and shop windows, in architecture and in gardens is altered in order to mediate human behaviour. For example, medical consultations with your GP take place in a clean, sound proofed room, with the right furniture and lighting and houses are commonly believed to sell more easily if the smells of freshly baked bread or coffee pervade.

The outdoor environment is consistent in its changeability. Seasons change and geographical location changes what is seen, smelt and heard. Clearly the outdoor environment experienced when skiing is very different to the one experienced in hill country walking activities in the UK. Some businesses try to reproduce the outdoor experience in the inside of the shop, perhaps erecting tents when selling outdoor pursuit goods and equipment or using an interesting mixture of blue and white colours, cold temperatures and the realistic sound and feel of snow to recreate a feeling of actual involvement with the mountain activity. This is then cleverly supported by alpine style food and services.

In the previous chapter an explanation of emotion was given and the relationship between emotions and triggers from the five senses was outlined. The environmental factors above can be used to trigger certain emotional responses and memories. Memories are themselves triggers for emotions, giving the same feeling as was felt at the time of the event which produced the memory.

Similarly, Attention Deficit and Hyperactivity Disorder (ADHD) sufferers find concentrating at a desk in a classroom very hard to achieve. However allowing the same education to be given whilst engaged in an outdoor activity can be far more successful. The emotional stimuli produced and the ability to be drawn back to the outdoor task allows learning to take place.

2.1 Being outside

The outdoor environment is characterised by:-

- large views of the sky
- a horizon
- changing seasons
- weather
- smells
- fresh air
- birdsong
- air movement felt against the skin
- sunlight (even through clouds)
- vibrant colours
- everyday activities of nature

For the purpose of discussing the outdoor environment in this book I have assumed that the location is rural or coastal and not too close to an urban setting. It is understood that a garden in a city may be a therapeutic space demonstrating seasons, colours and wildlife but it would not necessarily be able to offer the whole of the benefits due perhaps to traffic or air quality issues.

The characteristics of the outdoor environment given above stimulate human emotions and enhance cerebral functioning. Being outside “in the fresh air” is good for people. These effects can be seen in the increased need for sleep on an outdoor holiday caused by different and constant stimulations and activity, improved wellbeing and a better level of relaxation.

Exercise taken in a gym is clearly beneficial in terms of general fitness, weight management, cardiovascular and musculoskeletal health and improved mood. Exercise taken outside, however, improves wellbeing further when compared to the same exercise programme taken indoors. The outdoor environment stimulates an emotional response which enhances concentration and improves mood, thereby enhancing well being. This in turn increases motivation.

People often report that a sense of perspective is restored when they are reminded that days and seasons continue unchanged and that the universe is larger than their personal problems or difficulties.

Creativity is another important aspect of being human and some of the art inspired by the observation of nature is amongst the most powerful. This is often created whilst being outside and experiencing first hand the sights, sounds and smells. The emotionally triggered state of heightened awareness increases the ability to observe. How often is the experience of nature’s colours so vivid that it evokes the “they’d never believe it if you used that colour to paint it” response. The smell of cut grass brings up memories and their associated emotions to many people and life is richer for it. Sadly this may be an experience denied to those living in arid places or concrete cities. English scientists have shown that just as little as 5 minutes spent exercising outside can boost mood and self-esteem.

2.2 Outside and engaged

Just three hundred generations ago humans used to hunt and gather food and were nomadic. They evolved into farming communities and gained understanding of seasons and harvest which, when added to their knowledge of natural habitat and animal behaviour, enhanced their food options and therefore improved their health. The resilience of our ancestors is well demonstrated by the fact that the human race is still functional, albeit a little troubled in modern times. This involvement with the land continued from pre-history through to recent years with food production for the world still being land based.

2.3 Biophilia

In 1984 Wilson published his book called “Biophilia” and launched his Biophilia Hypothesis. It expounded that, despite the divorce of most from the land based activities, people still

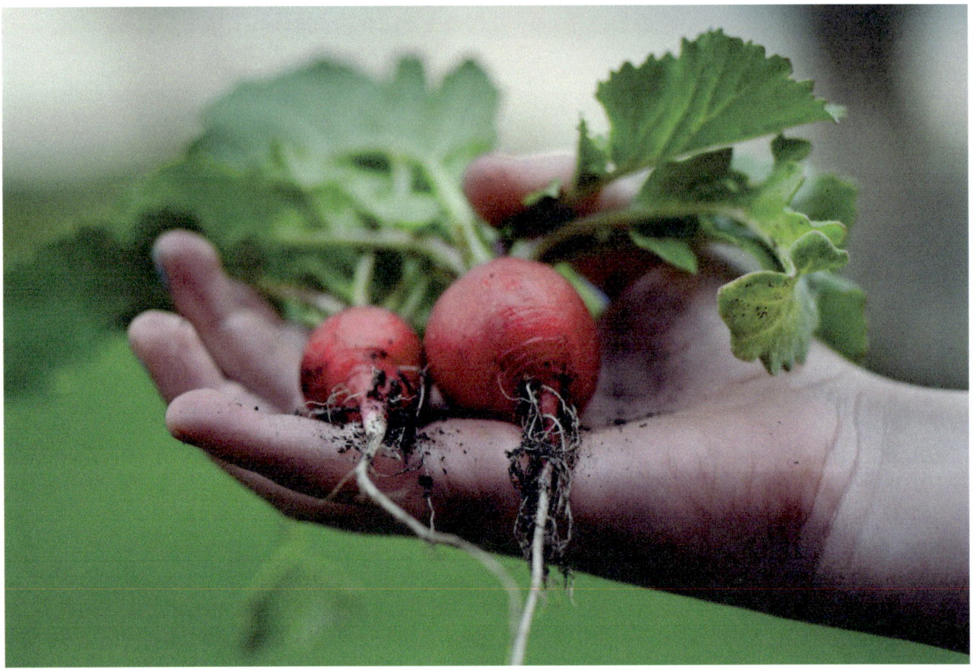

Image 3: Growing things with purpose

wanted to grow things and be engaged with an agricultural aspect, no matter how small. This is fairly well demonstrated throughout the United Kingdom with a passion for gardens, growing flowers, fruit and vegetables, with allotments and even window boxes and hanging baskets seen frequently in built up areas. The Biophilia Hypothesis was well tested over many years and was taken further in 2007 when various scientists backed a theory stating that, despite human evolution, mankind remained focussed on life and life processes. The sight of cut grass drying for hay is known to excite feelings of satisfaction in people, whilst growing vegetables and flowers for specific purposes is known to address mental health and social issues. Working with animals and animal husbandry have also been researched and found to be successful in improving human wellbeing.

Horticulture, agriculture and animal husbandry all harness the benefits of the outdoor environment and add the biophilic activities of "growing things with purpose" to enhance the feeling of well-being produced. Outdoor activities, those which are exercise, experience or adventure based, have also been introduced and studied. The positive effects of outdoor activity on physical, mental and emotional health, human behaviour and learning have been harnessed internationally for some years. Many countries started using outdoor pursuits to improve general fitness, self-confidence, health and resilience in the 1960s. Then, because of the recognised benefits, the outdoor activity or pursuits programmes were included in mainstream educational provision. Programmes were also seen to assist people with disadvantage to successfully modify behaviour and improve overall health and wellbeing.

2.4 Outdoor therapy and its history

Outdoor therapy as a term is high level, generic and used as an umbrella term. Internationally outdoor therapy encompasses a range of therapeutic activities including:-

- Adventure and Wilderness therapy
- Horticulture and Agriculture based therapy
- Outdoor pursuits with therapeutic application
- Nature and Environmental based therapy

In the USA the provision of outdoor therapy, particularly as adventure and wilderness therapy, is well established with most states having centres. Similarly most states have at least one Barn Centre where horses are used to positively affect human health. The American programmes for military veterans are extensive and range from free-climbing to fly fishing. Fly fishing is an excellent example of an outdoor pursuit or activity which produces grounding or mindfulness. Horse riding is another. The first international conference of adventure therapy was held in Australia in 1967 whilst the first international conference of HETI was held in Paris in 1974. It is clear that nothing that is described here

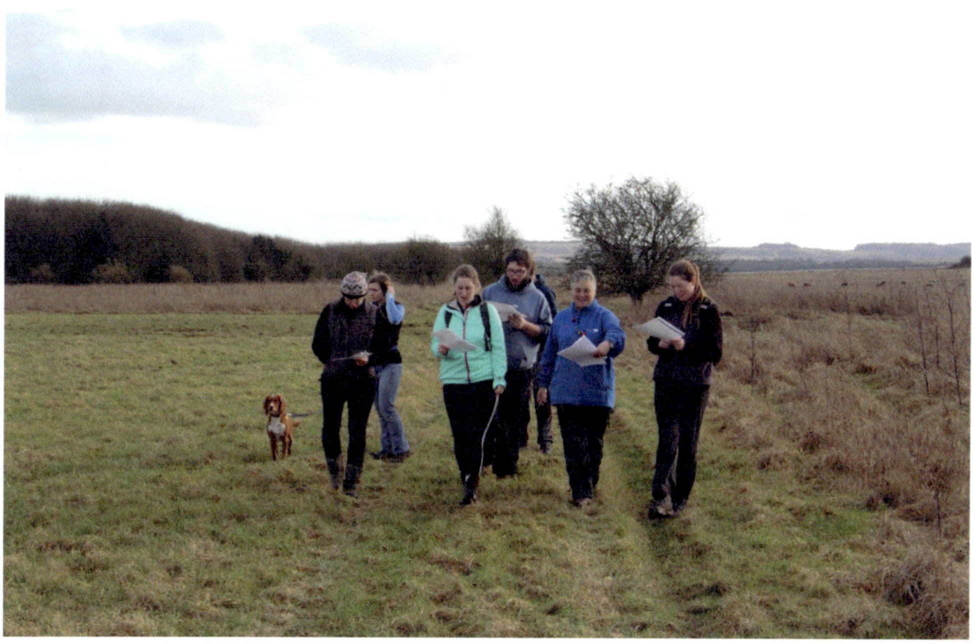

Image 4: Group learning to map read

is particularly new or untested, even if many in UK are hitherto unaware of the potential benefits.

Case study 2

Marion self-referred on the advice of her GP. She is a 32 year old lady with a colourful past and a current addiction to alcohol. She frequently feels lonely and has been diagnosed with a borderline personality disorder. This has led to the use of alcohol as self medication. Marion can become very anxious in all manner of situations and feels at odds with the world. She is known for outbursts of anger. Marion has had several partners but no children and is currently living alone, on benefits, in a city centre flat.

As a child, Marion enjoyed horses and horse riding and was interested to hear from her GP that Gul could offer this activity. She arrived in a very stressed state with colourful clothing and immediately needed to have a cigarette following the journey to Gul, during which she and the friend who had driven her here had become lost.

The assessment showed that Marion would benefit from being outside for physical activity thereby helping her to sleep and fill time without thinking about alcohol. Coming to the yard would benefit Marion by giving a sense of belonging and value and, as she had previous horse experience, it was suggested she joined as a supported helper.

Funding for this was discussed and Marion was in receipt of Personal Independence Payments which she would use to pay to attend.

It was felt that Marion would benefit from being enabled to succeed, whether this was in relationship with others, attending work on a regular basis or learning new things. She would benefit from increasing her self awareness, noticing how she felt about situations, learning to recognise her feelings as well as the feelings of others and making appropriate responses to them.

It was discussed that noticing anger before it became out of hand would be a useful skill that she might work on. There was no need to educate Marion, nor particularly to focus on her communication skills. Marion's physical ability was good enough, but psychological oversight of her supported volunteering would be appropriate.

Marion was assisted to find public transport solutions to her travelling and decided to attend two mornings a week. She would help with horse care on both mornings and on one of them have a short session of riding with goals for mindfulness and relaxation. This was therefore likely to be a bareback session. The forms were duly completed and Marion commenced attendance.

Every so often Marion would simply not arrive. It soon became clear that this was after a drinking session the night before. The team helped Marion to understand what precipitated these and to look at the consequences of drinking, these very simple observational exercises reduced the frequency of non-attendance considerably.

Marion said "I really love coming here, I feel like I'm part of the team" and started to take on more and more roles and responsibilities. The senior therapist talked with Marion about this pointing out this was a pattern seen in her life where her natural competency got ahead of her, causing her to take on too much when feeling positive, only to drop it all when feeling less good and therefore letting people down.

Marion was encouraged to try less hard to please everyone and to discover how to become more resilient by pacing herself.

Nine months on, Marion is still attending the Centre, is greeted by name and valued as a useful member of the horse care team.

Chapter 3

Horses, the extra factor

3.0 Why horses?

People have been associated with horses for thousands of years. People have worked with them, hunted from them, travelled and transported using them and gone to war with them. Some even eat them.

Winston Churchill did not consider himself a horseman, but nonetheless observed that "there is something about the outside of a horse that is good for the inside of a man".

Today some go so far as to say that there is something about the whole of a horse that is good for the wholeness of a person. This strong and historic bond between man and horse can still be seen through the many contacts people choose to have with horses today. Horses continue to provoke strong reactions in people; love, hate and fear to name but three.

3.1 The physical effect

Horses are large (usually) and powerful animals, warm to touch and able to carry humans. Even the smaller breeds native to UK, such as Shetland and the Welsh Section A, were used to carry adults across rough moorland. It is only comparatively recently that these breeds have been used as childrens' ponies. Many readers will agree that the temperaments of these breeds are not always suited to this role.

Riding a horse gives physical exercise as well as associated emotional responses. The husbandry requirements of keeping horses leads to ongoing physical exercise. Various papers have studied the calorie usage when engaged in horse related activities and the rough rule is:-

- 100 calories used per hour of gentle hacking
- 200 calories used per hour of vigorous mucking out
- 400 calories used per hour of riding cross country with purpose

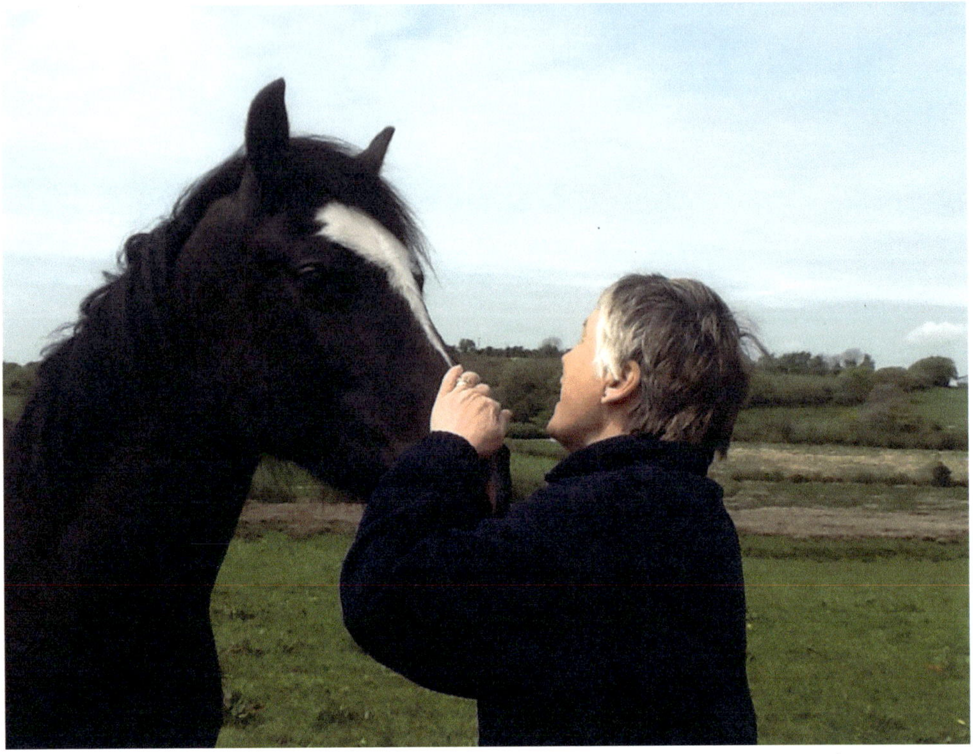

Image 5: Having a chat

In addition to the above the horse has a very specific physical effect on a human. When sitting on a horse at walk the movement passively reproduces in the rider the same movements that would occur during healthy, active walking.

To achieve normal walking, a healthy human pelvis, lower spine and hips need to move freely in all three planes of orientation of pitch, roll and yaw. Pitch is the movement required to bend a person over to touch their toes. Roll is the movement which allows the sliding of a hand down the outer edge of a leg to the knee. Yaw is the movement of rotating the front of the pelvis to point left or right of straight ahead. Only two animals have this effect on human movement: horses and pigs. In general, despite the undisputed intelligence of pigs, riding horses is considered more practical and is certainly more popular!

3.2 Horses and emotions

Horse intelligence varies across a spectrum as it does for any animal, but the small cerebrum of the horse brain means little logical reasoning takes place. The horse functions mostly at the limbic, or emotional, level of the brain. They don't reason but rather react through instinct and the herd response protects them as prey animals. The brain stem functions are those that keep horses and people alive and include basic functions such as breathing, swallowing and reflex withdrawal from pain. The limbic area of the brain is located next to it and lies between the brain stem and the cerebral cortex. The limbic system is the area of the brain where emotions, or feelings, arise. Many people are not aware of their emotions and may even actively suppress them to avoid embarrassment. Working with horses, however, can cause people's emotions to be displayed strongly and a therapist can use this catalytic effect of the horse's impact on emotion to help the rider to understand and explain to them what is at play in a situation.

3.3 Horses and reflection

The horse lives at this emotional level without the verbal or written word. They communicate non-verbally and are non-judgemental. They neither notice nor care how a person looks, they just notice how the person feels, or put in another way, what emotion the person is really feeling. They notice whether emotion is displayed or hidden and some horses can be visibly unsettled by incongruity in a person, i.e. by a person behaving in a way that is at odds with how they actually feel. Someone stating that they aren't afraid, whilst feeling fear, can cause some horses to show dislike or distrust of that person by laying their ears flat or tail swishing. These horses are of great value in therapy settings.

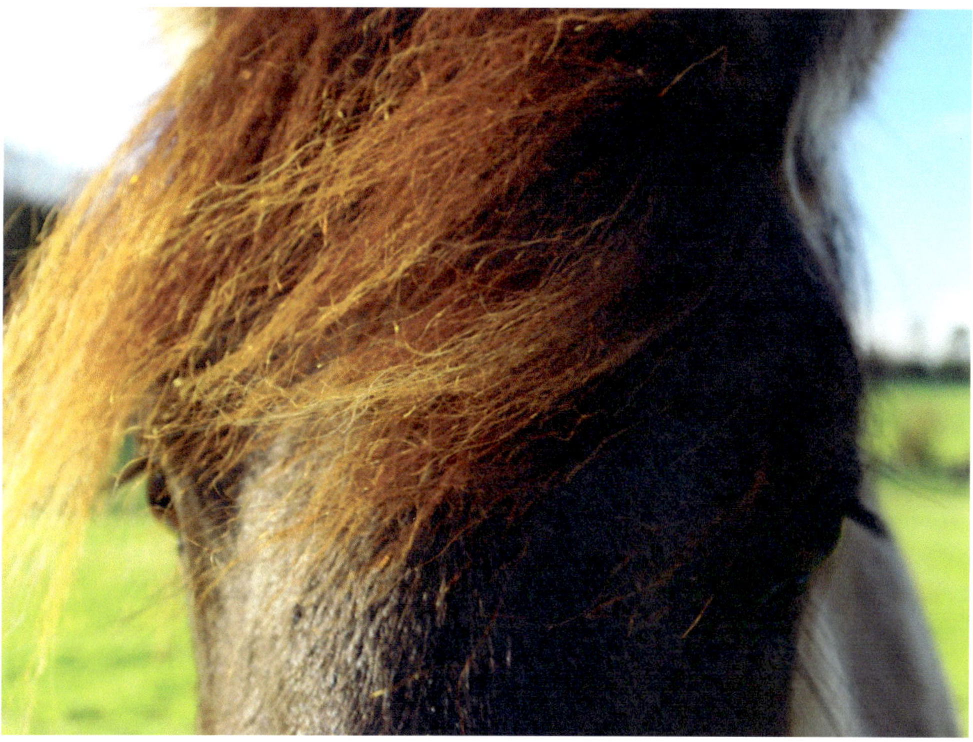

Image 6: Through the eyes of the horse

Other horses, when faced with a human exhibiting anxious humour, will display fear in response to the underlying anxiety and so show the therapist the strong emotion of the person, whether the person recognises or acknowledges this anxiety or not. This process is called reflection and a reflective horse, one which readily shows the person's real feelings, is again an excellent partner to have in a therapeutic intervention.

The reason the horse reacts in this way follows from the herd response to danger and other emotions. When danger presents a herd will exhibit the "one startles and all react" behaviour, as seen in preyed upon animals. The horse picks up on the emotions of other horses and, usefully for therapy, the emotion of humans and responds to it in a way that keeps the horse safe and engaged in their herd.

3.4 Horse character and personality

Horses have characters and personalities just as people and other animals do. The personalities of horses are covered by several schools of thought. Most agree that a horse will have two aspects to their personality, a dominant one and a less dominant. The dominant aspect is mostly displayed and is partly mediated by the less dominant one. Once stressed the horse reverts fully to the dominant aspect only.

One well known classification of horse personality uses such terms as:-

- social
- fearful
- challenging
- aloof

The above gives rise to pairs of personality aspects e.g. social and aloof and so on.

There are different descriptions by various authors available and readers should become familiar with whichever categorisation furthers their own understanding. This will also aid communication between the therapy team. The thing to note is that horses do have personalities and these need to be taken into consideration when choosing which horse to use in therapy.

In addition to the dominant and less dominant aspects of their personality the following add their effect to horse behaviour:-

- gender – whether mare, stallion or gelding
- age
- life experiences
- breed

Some breed characteristics pre-dispose to certain behaviours. For example, Welsh Ponies and Cobs can be "sharp" i.e. highly reactive, whilst Shetland Ponies can be challenging and New Forest Ponies are typically cleverer than the average horse.

In addition to the above, the horse is an outside animal and the seasons' effect on their hormones, the quality of grass and their general wellbeing will affect their behaviour on a daily basis.

Horses form relationships and this again endears them to people. Most like companionship and physical contact and are happy to share these with people as well as with other horses. In horses with a predominantly social character these aspects of companionship and physical contact are easily available to humans.

Horses do not seek to please, unlike dogs. They just accept a person into their view of the herd and give them a hierarchy rating. This is another useful equine behaviour helpful in therapy when treating people with issues relating to with self-confidence, bullying and self-assertion.

3.5 Horses in therapeutic intervention

The usual triangle depicting relationships within a therapeutic intervention is shown in Fig. 5.

The triangle of Fig. 5 is used in every routine, room based therapeutic intervention. A therapist selects an appropriate intervention from their "toolbox" which is covered in Chapter 4. The intervention is chosen to make the desired improvement in the physical, mental or emotional health, human behaviour, general wellbeing or education of the person receiving the therapy. The tool used could be a specific form of psychological therapy such as Cognitive Behavioural Therapy or a specific tool from within that area of work.

Fig. 5: Therapeutic relationships triangle

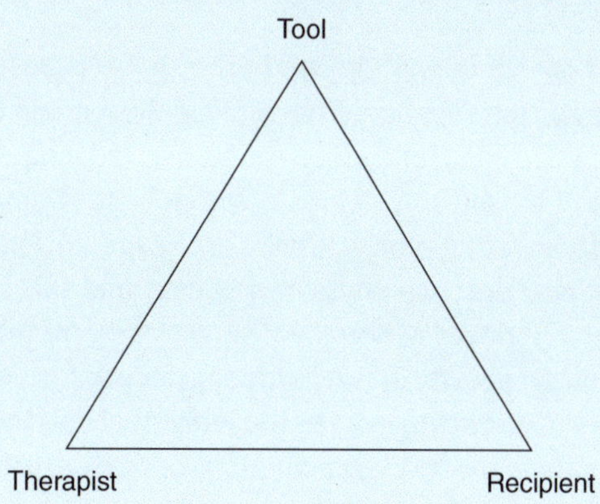

3.5.1 Activity based therapy

In therapy such as play, art or music, an activity is added. This is used to add to the effect of the therapy on offer. Therapy can still be offered at various levels and, at the lower level, the activity such as dance or painting is a therapeutic activity simply facilitated by the coach or therapy assistant. At a higher level a therapist may be drawing on cues from the person and enable the recipient to move on.

In the case of a physiotherapy intervention the physiotherapist, with knowledge of the underlying physical need, will choose a specific activity or exercise to work on with the patient. They will work on this with due regard for the difficulty the patient feels, but with progress towards the goals in mind.

Fig. 6: Therapeutic relationships square

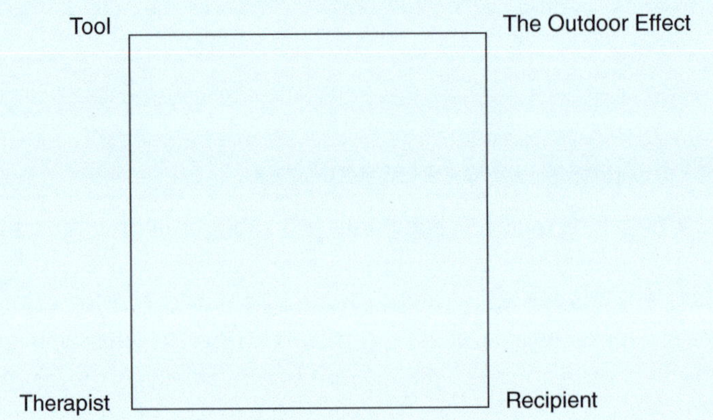

3.5.2 Outdoor therapy

In generic outdoor therapy the relationship changes as shown in Fig. 7.

The outdoor effect has now come into play and an activity is chosen that will enhance the outcome of the therapeutic intervention. The activity chosen will clearly have an effect. A bicycle, for example, could be used for cycling, navigation, adventure or building an outdoor pursuits skill. It can also be used to produce a whole host of emotions such as exhilaration, fatigue and frustration. Using a bicycle may evoke memories and the emotions associated with them. It will also produce physical tiredness and this sooner than expected as the average general fitness reduces nationally. This is clearly complex and outdoor pursuits Instructors are aware that an activity in the outdoors can produce emotion and subsequent behaviour which may need managing to keep the individual and the group safe. The bicycle itself, however, is inanimate and won't voice opinions or react to any behaviour of the therapist or participant, nor indeed to the weather.

Fig. 7: Therapeutic relationships crown

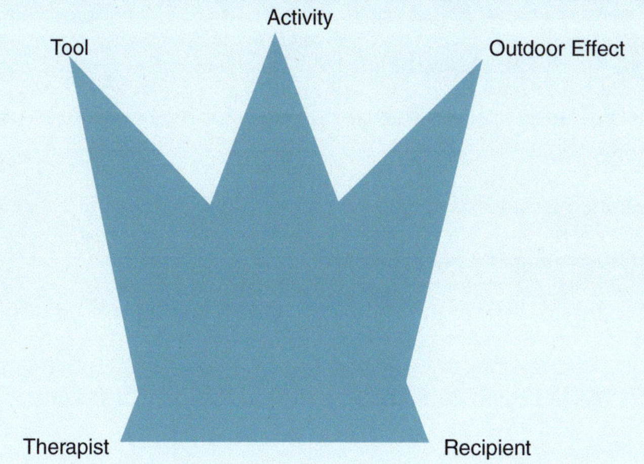

In outdoor therapy the therapist will choose the combination of activity and difficulty that produces the best opportunity to progress towards the goals of the recipient of therapy.

3.5.3 Horse based therapy

In horse based therapy there is a further, complex dimension added which can be shown in Fig. 8 below. In this field of therapy the inanimate objects, e.g. bikes and climbing walls are replaced by a horse.

Fig. 8: Therapeutic relationships crown, 4 point

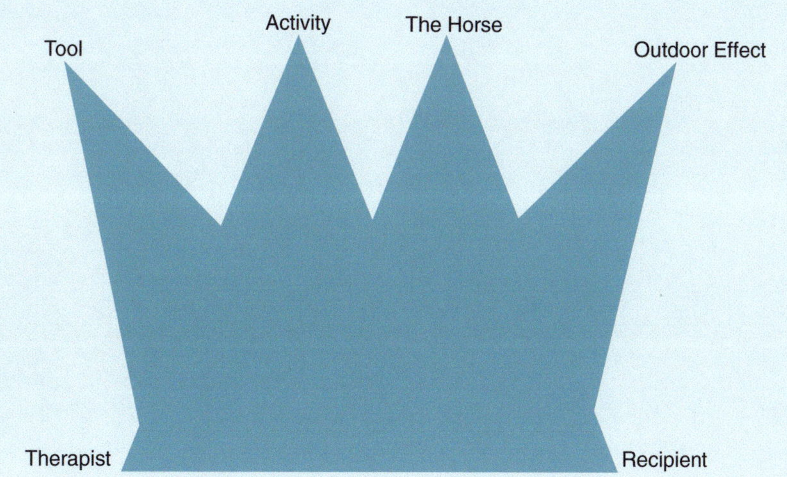

This extra dimension is rarely understood by people without horse knowledge and yet it is essential for understanding the impact of horse based therapy.

It can be seen that the therapist now needs to:-

- select the programme or tool which is appropriate for the recipient to use to work towards the goals
- select a horse which is suitable
- select a good choice of horse based activity
- decide whether to add the enhanced emotional and physical stimulation of working outside or not
- ensure they are the best available therapist for the recipient's session
- timetable the intervention

When horse based therapy is really effective the therapist moves from leading the therapy to the role of interpreter. Their role now is to interpret the interactions taking place between the horse and person. The relationship between person and horse is now the main aspect in play and so becomes the therapeutic intervention. Some call this zone "seeing the world differently through the eyes of the horse" and is shown pictorially in Fig. 9.

Fig. 9: Therapeutic relationships crown 4 point version 2

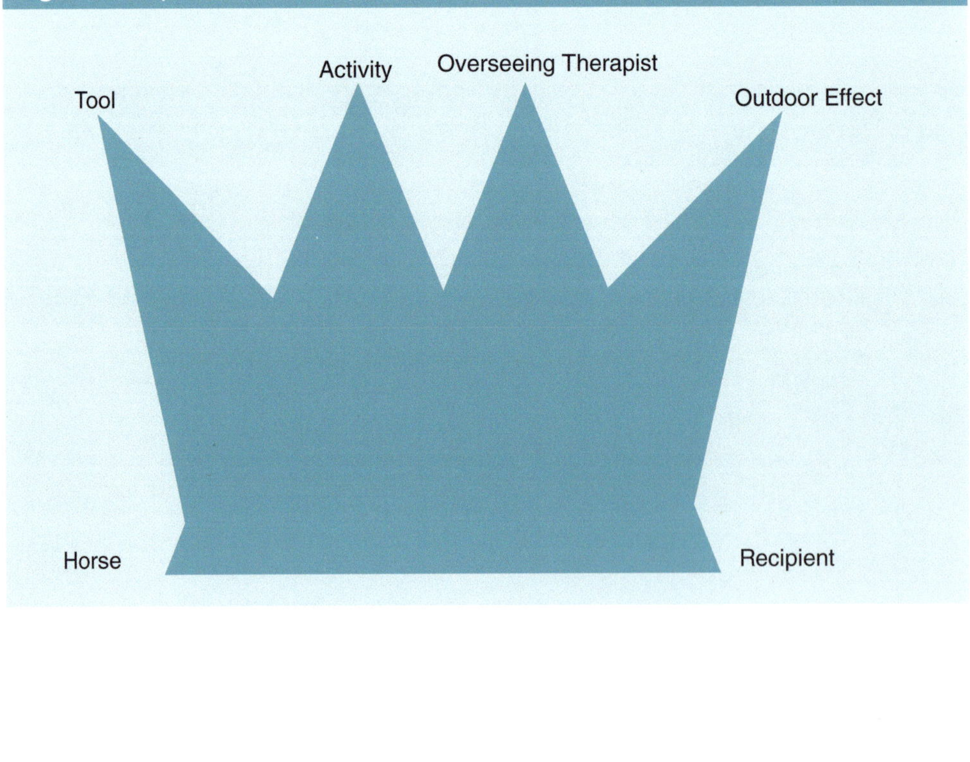

3.6 Choice of Horse

The choice of the horse is so important that it appears in the considerations area of the horse based therapy matrix. The choice needs to take into consideration that the outdoor effect will have an effect on the horse's behaviour as well as the person's behaviour. Whilst cycling on a windy day may be more physically demanding, a windy day with a sharp horse on spring grass would be unlikely to produce a calm session if that was what was intended.

It is hoped that the progression through the preceding pages has given the essential background in which the choice of the horse is now understood.

The choice of the therapy depends on what a centre has available and the ability to provide for an individual can rest on this alone. If a centre does not have a suitable horse the potential recipient should be advised to look elsewhere.

Using a reflective horse can be useful to ensure the emotions voiced by the recipient (or their carer on their behalf) are confirmed as part of the assessment process.

The choice of the horse for an anxious person to ride is unlikely to be one that is fearful or reflective. They are unlikely to work well with a sharp horse either. An aloof horse would be a good choice for starting the process as such an animal won't react as strongly to the person's fear. A social horse could also be a good choice as their constant interactions and quickly formed relationships can distract the person from their anxiety.

For ground based intervention the choice can change again. If the goal for the recipient is to feel less fear then observing the behaviour of a reflective horse during ground work with them would act as a useful indicator of their own progress.

The therapist always has the option of proceeding initially without a horse if using a horse as well as outdoor stimulation is too great to manage. An activity such as stable or field management will be equally purposeful and effective but less complicated.

If the session is one in which the movement of the horse is the critical factor to bringing an improvement, the therapist will need to be clear what they are looking for on behalf of an individual.

The movement of the horse in walk moves the rider's pelvis through three planes. The warmth of the horse ridden bareback causes relaxation thereby allowing an improved range of movement. The therapist should be able to choose a horse that provides more side to side, more front to back or more rotational movement when needed in order to be most effective. Designing a course for a session which works on the rein and size of the circle to further increase the range of movement will also improve the outcome.

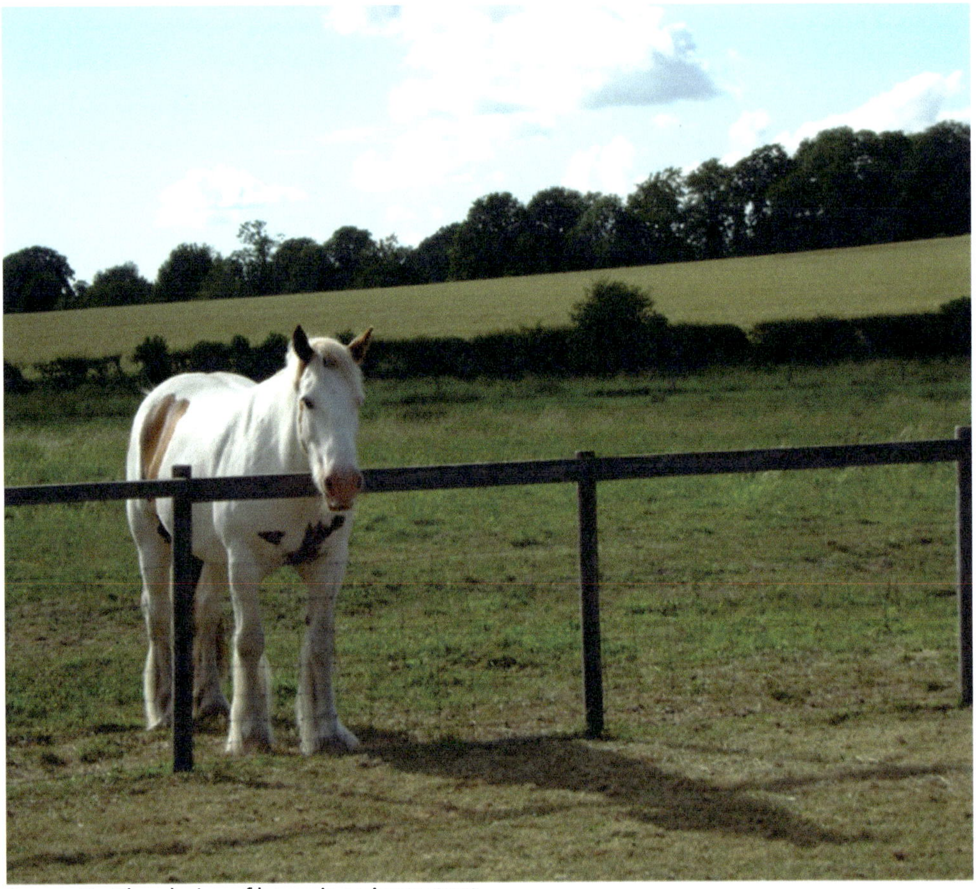

Image 7: The choice of horse is so important

When asking a physiotherapist why she thought this was the most powerful intervention she had ever used for low back pain the reply was that a physiotherapist could only work in two planes at once but the horse had an effect in three simultaneously. The shapes walked by the horse improves the effect still further.

An adult with cerebral palsy may need a quiet, non-reflective, short legged, stable, load carrying horse whose movement is straight and regular with minimal lateral effect. Whereas an adult attending a physiotherapist led session for improving low back pain may need something quite different with specific movements in the horse's gait needed to maximise the benefit of the session.

In this chapter I do not intend to teach a centre how to provide therapeutic interventions. Rather the aim is to show the full breadth of applications which could be used within any centre. In order to provide more of this work a centre would need staff with the relevant qualifications together with suitable horses and space.

Case study 3

Mike is an ex-soldier, now aged 50. He came to the Level 3 Centre on the advice of his GP. He had been a Senior Non-Commissioned Officer in an infantry unit and had had several active tours in Afghanistan and Iraq. Mike had symptoms of Post Traumatic Stress Disorder but this had not been formally diagnosed. The symptoms might also have fitted Generalised Anxiety Disorder. He was alerted, had recurring nightmares and some intrusive thoughts but was well enough to manage a job. This job, however, required very little contact with people. He found mixing with people very difficult.

He felt his relationship with his new partner was struggling. His ex-wife had left him because of his behaviour and anger. Mike needed to understand what was going on and it was decided that walking was the best therapy. The action of moving left foot, right foot, left foot is similar to the basis of the Eye Movement Desensitisation and Reprogramming (EMDR) treatment. The discovery of EMDR came from recognition of the thought processing work done by people whilst walking.

CBT was chosen as the intervention and was used during a walking activity. It was noted that this still fit ex-infantry soldier was faster walking uphill than the therapist working with him and the therapist soon learned to ask complex questions at the bottom of the hill so that they could merely listen during the climb! The real trigger which fed into the recurring nightmare had been one specific incident under fire in Afghanistan when a child casualty had reminded him of a niece in the United Kingdom. The therapist approached this with him and finally a date was set when the entire scenario would be revisited. As in most cases like this, Mike did not "remember" the incident he "relived it". Mike could describe the strength of wind, the smell on the wind, the direction of the wind, the light, the call sign of the mortar unit and all of this in great detail. Using Memory Addressing Techniques the session was gone through and Mike reported a reduction in nightmares with immediate effect. He found the nightmares only returned at times of stress and came only occasionally to the centre for times of walking therapy with refreshing of understanding or coping strategies. Mike's relationship did not survive but his ability to work did and he felt life was as successful as he could hope at the moment.

Chapter 4

The matrix expanded

4.0 Areas of application

The concept of using a matrix was introduced in chapter one and now its headings and use requires fuller explanation.

The matrix is shown again below

Fig.10

Level	Considerations	Areas of applications									
Therapeutic interventions offered		Possibilities									

If the matrix for generic outdoor therapy is considered it could be expected that outdoor activities in which therapy could be offered would be those currently provided by outdoor pursuit providers and such activities would be entered into the Areas of Application as seen in the above figure.

There is no order or priority implied by an activity's position in the list. Priority can only be assigned on an individual basis based on potential usefulness for an individual's therapy. The lists given in this book are not to be taken as complete or definitive. A list of all the possible applications could not be offered as these will change with geography and are constantly evolving.

The whole process of using a matrix is to enable therapists or therapy teams:-

- to be clear about what they offer
- to inform potential recipients and their families
- to inform potential purchasers such as schools and social workers
- to see what other types of provision people could be offered elsewhere
- to refresh the applications and therapeutic interventions offered as provision changes over time.

Now that the Areas of Application are displayed for outdoor therapy it can be seen that horse related therapy is one part of a large whole.

Areas of Application																				
Agriculture	Abseiling	Climbing	Cycling	Camping	Countryside Skills	Canoe and Kayaking	Ecology	Exped. and Adventure	Forestry	Horticulture	Horse Based Activity	Nav. and Orienteering	Running	Sailing and Windsurfing	Surfing	Walking	Wilderness	Volunteering	Work Experience	OTHER

Fig. 11: Areas of Application in outdoor therapy

4.1 Therapeutic interventions

An understanding of the range of therapeutic interventions routinely on offer throughout the world in Outdoor Therapy can be summarised in eight, high level groupings. The types of therapies are offered across the range of physical, mental and emotional health, general wellbeing, improved human behaviour and alternative education.

These are:-

- Outdoor activity for physical health and general well being
- Belonging through purposeful activity
- Enabling success
- Self-awareness
- Education
- Communication
- Physical therapies for maintenance, rehabilitation and treatment
- Psychological therapies

These headings are the entries in the "therapeutic interventions offered" section of the therapy matrix as seen in Fig. 10 above.

The therapeutic interventions shown have not been chosen because they only work in a horse based setting but because they are known to work.

They have the added benefit of being widely used and accepted.

The temptation to create new approaches is better avoided until this field of work is better understood and more widely available at its simplest level. In its simplest form it can be the provision of a recognised therapeutic intervention delivered in an outdoor setting.

It cannot be assumed that successful programmes from other countries can be directly imported to the UK. One lesson learned from health and education is that not all successful American programmes can be directly imported to UK. As a minimum the language used needs to be reviewed so it synchronises with the "British, therefore different" way of doing things.

4.2 Levels of therapy

The level of therapy offered by different centres will be varied and dependent on many factors. Rather than leaving the perception of capability unsupported, a provider should be asked to give an overview of what level they can offer. This is best done using the system shown below. The levels are ranked 1 to 3 where level 1 is the lowest level of capability and level 3 the highest. It is suggested that the following guide is adopted.

Level 1	**Therapy Assistant level of provision.** The provision at this centre is able to follow a plan devised and supervised by a therapist, teacher, social worker or carer, who may not be present during the session. An example would be of volunteering for well being
Level 2	**Therapist level of provision.** The provision at this centre is able to devise and supervise a plan in a particular area of expertise or qualification. An example would be a physiotherapy based intervention for physical rehabilitation
Level 3	**Full Therapeutic range of provision provided by a team approach.** The provision at this centre is able to devise and supervise programmes to assist physical, mental, emotional and behavioural issues through a highly qualified team with sufficient experience in all of these areas.

Fig. 12: Levels of capability within outdoor therapy

A Level 1 centre would not be able to assess the individual. It would be able to follow a plan agreed with the responsible worker for the person. A Level 1 centre would need to be working under the supervision of a more qualified organisation.

A Level 2 or 3 centre would have the ability to assess an individual, devise a therapeutic course and manage it through. A Level 2 or 3 centre would be able to look for wider issues, such as whether there was external support for change, or if there are other aspects of care which may affect the hoped for outcomes.

4.3 Considerations in therapy

The section on consideration is shown in Fig. 10 in level in Fig. 10 above. The considerations were explained to be the overarching rules and external factors that could affect the provision for the individual entering or considering therapy.

The rules and facilities of a particular centre will affect the therapeutic offer before these further considerations are applied. The considerations given next are directly linked to the person considering attending.

There are five main considerations which will affect the provision offered:-

- age of the person (or age group if adult)
- disadvantage or disadvantages to be addressed
- severity of the condition or conditions
- staffing ratio likely to be required eg group session or 1:1
- home situation

Example Outdoor Therapy Matrix

Name:	Therapy ass/Coach:	Date:

Level	Considerations
1	Age Disadvantage and Severity 1:1 in school hours

Areas of Application / **Possibilities available**

Therapeutic Interventions	Agriculture	Abseiling	Climbing	Cycling	Camping	Countryside Skills	Canoe and Kayaking	Ecology	Exped and Adventure	Forestry	Horticulture	Horse Based Activity	Nav. and Orienteering	Running	Sailing and Windsurfing	Surfing	Walking	Wilderness	Volunteering	Work Experience	OTHER
Activity for physical health and wellbeing																					
Belonging and value through purposeful activity																					
Enabling Success																					
Self-Awareness																					
Education																					
Communication																					
Occupational and Physio therapy, treatment, maintenance, rehabilitation																					
Psychological therapies and counselling																					

Fig. 13: outdoor therapy matrix

Whilst it may seem obvious it is worth being clear that the person attending needs to be safe to be involved in the activity suggested and that their disability or disadvantage will neither preclude their participation nor make it unsafe.

When the type of outdoor therapy chosen is to be horse based the choice of horse becomes another consideration on the matrix as shown below.

The multiplicity of factors can be seen on the matrix and the number of possibilities for therapy for an individual are shown by the number of boxes in the possibilities section. For the matrix above these number 160

Example of using a matrix

An example of using the outdoor therapy matrix. Let us consider a course of action for a teenager with severe Autistic Spectrum Disorder (ASD) and challenging behaviour being referred to a centre by their Social Worker. The referral was for supported work experience.

In this scenario the reader should imagine their centre to be an Outdoor Therapy Centre (OTC) with more than just horse based work but not offering the full range of outdoor activities. The centre has judged itself capable of delivering to level 1 and has all proper measures in place for provision.

The Outdoor Therapy matrix of the centre is likely to look like the one shown below and shaded areas are those which not offered.

The considerations show that 1 to 1 staffing is only available during the school day in term time and not at weekends or holidays.

The matrix shown allows discussion to take place and as the challenging behaviour is mild and rarely seen in 1 to 1 sessions with no danger to the teenager or others, it is decided an on site assessment is appropriate.

It is not expected that all possibilities in a matrix will be offered.

The offer to an individual should be enough to enable staff to deliver interesting and safe sessions for a young person as described above.

The X marked squares would be a good initial offer.

The last decision regarding the offer is who would hold responsibility for the case. In this case, as the centre is Level 1, this clearly remains with the Social Worker. Agreement needs to be reached about what can and cannot be managed at the centre in terms of challenging behaviour.

Example Outdoor Therapy Matrix

Name:	Therapy ass/Coach:	Date:

Level	Considerations
1	Age Disadvantage and Severity 1:1 in school hours

Therapeutic Interventions	Agriculture	Abseiling	Climbing	Cycling	Camping	Countryside Skills	Canoe and Kayaking	Ecology	Exped. and Adventure	Forestry	Horticulture	Horse Based Activity	Nav. and Orienteering	Running	Sailing and Windsurfing	Surfing	Walking	Wilderness	Volunteering	Work Experience	OTHER
Activity for physical health and wellbeing																					
Belonging and value through purposeful activity																					
Enabling Success																					
Self-Awareness																					
Education																					
Communication																					
Occupational and Physio therapy, treatment, maintenance, rehabilitation																					
Psychological therapies and counselling																					

(Header above the area columns: **Areas of Application**; header above the intervention rows: **Possibilities available**)

Fig. 14: Example Outdoor Therapy Centre matrix

The centre could offer a trial with an agreement that the teenager would be referred back to the Social Worker to affect a change in any behaviour that the centre is finding difficult and consider ending the placement if this is not successful.

The centre could signpost to other provisions if available.

4.4 The horse based therapy matrix

Fig. 15 shows a completed matrix for horse based therapy. It can be seen that the therapeutic interventions have not changed from those used in the generic matrix but the previously seen areas of application relevant for outdoor therapy have been replaced with purely equine ones.

The areas of application now reflect a range of horse based activities suited to use in therapy.

Once again this is neither definitive nor exhaustive. It could be changed by anyone as needed. Nor does any centre need to offer all the possibilities shown here, just the ones their therapy team, surroundings and horses can provide.

The considerations box, “previously blue yellow in colour”, now has an extra factor to consider, that of the choice of horse as detailed above.

4.5 Therapeutic interventions expanded and explained

4.5.1 Outdoor activity for physical health and wellbeing

This is the simplest intervention and the one with the most widespread application.

The understanding of the benefit of outdoor activity on physical and mental health and well- being is growing. Local Authorities in the UK, now hosts to Public Health departments, are leading on designing programmes for physical activity for all ages. Country-wide, local authority led partnerships are commissioning and providing the programmes and this work is driven partly by the rising numbers of obese adults and children and partly by increasing numbers of mental health problems.

There is an array of swimming programmes, slimming clubs on prescription, walking clubs, forest schools and many other healthy lifestyle provisions being delivered across the nation. They may use private, public or third sector providers and some attract charitable funding. Many of these are already delivered in the outdoor environment.

Outdoor activity for physical health and wellbeing can be provided by any centre.

Generic Horse Based Therapy Template

Name:	Therapist:	Date:

Level	Considerations	Areas of Application																				
Not spec-ified	Age Disadvantage Severity 1:1 or group Horse (s)	Field Management	Bareback riding	Back Riding	Competition	Countryside Skills	Driving	Ethogram work	Ground work	Horse Agility	Horse Care	Connection	Long Lining	Riding as a sport	Riding with goals	Stable Management	Training the horse	Vaulting	Volunteering	Wheelchair work	Work Experience	Other
Therapeutic Interventions		**Possibilities available**																				
Outdoor Activity for physical health and wellbeing																						
Belonging and value through purposeful activity																						
Enabling Success																						
Self-Awareness																						
Education																						
Communication																						
Occupational/physio therapy treatment/rehab/maintenance																						
Psychological therapies and counselling																						

Fig 15: Horse based therapy matrix

Whilst people have a need to be busy and have purpose in their lives, the current attachment to digital technology and the intensity of modern day living are not necessarily good for health.

Outdoor activity often requires people attending to turn electronic devices off so allowing reduced levels of stimulation and increased emotional processing during activities. Turning off the devices also ensures the ability to communicate and form relationships is maintained and developed.

Outdoor activity does not have to be part of a gym type programme, it can cover a wide range of levels of exercise suited to the age, ability and fitness of the participants. The benefit is not necessarily derived from physical exertion but from the effect of being outside and engaged in something which is not purely sedentary.

Outdoor activity may well improve physical health by increasing fitness, enabling weight control and reducing the risks of illness such as diabetes, osteoarthritis and cardiac disease. These are important benefits but there is also a positive effect on mental well being. Being outdoors and engaged in activity allows the brain to process thoughts, process events and rest, thereby improving sleep, mood and concentration.

4.5.2 Belonging and value through purposeful activity

There are several well known and often used psychological tools which show the progression of needs common to all humans from being safe and warm with food and drink available, up to education, close relationship, social interaction and purpose. Maslow's Hierarchy of Need is one such tool.

Belonging may be taken for granted by those who have families, work in a team or who belong to a club of some kind but for others, particularly the disadvantaged, turning up somewhere they are greeted by name can be very affirming.

People in employment hopefully feel they are involved in purposeful activity whilst at work. At the very least employment allows earning and self worth. School students and unemployed adults do not have this route to value open to them and have to ensure their days feel purposeful. Clearly this presents problems for the non academic student required to be in a school setting.

If day time activities for any one person do not bring a sense of belonging or value or purpose then evenings and weekends need to be used for this instead.

The provision of this therapeutic intervention needs to pay attention to the use of the word "purposeful". Horses give rise to unending amounts of purposeful and repeated activity from grooming them to cleaning tack, sweeping yards and feeding to name but a few. The horse's need for husbandry is an integral part of their therapeutic role.

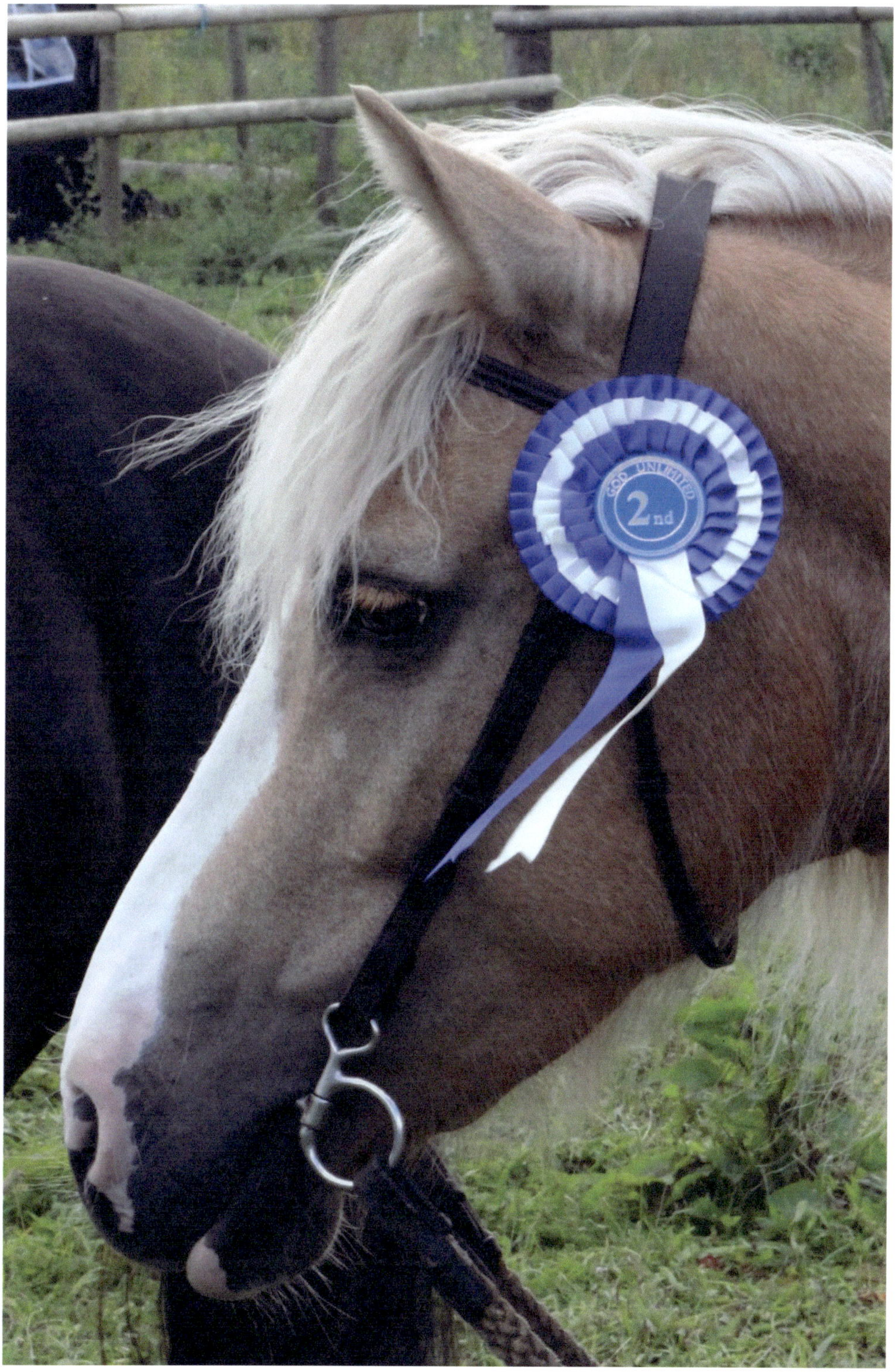

Image 8: A rosette as a marker of success

Farms provide a similar spectrum of purposeful activity which is why agriculture appears on the outdoor therapy matrix but clearly the added value of interaction and relationship with horses brings extra benefit.

Again this therapeutic intervention could be provided by any mainstream riding centre.

4.5.3 Enabling success

The definitions of success include words and phrases such as achievement, accomplishment and realisation of goals, results wanted or aims hoped for. The concept of succeeding is central to life itself.

The meeting of a basic need, such as finding fresh water, counts as a success at the most important level to any animal, that of survival. Not all successes have to be so important.

Successes, however small, lead to self-belief and the understanding that the person matters and can have a life with purpose. Successes encourage and give something to build on, so helping people to move on with their lives. Some self-confidence is essential for successful living and is developed through self-belief, which in turn is developed through success.

Enabling success can be achieved by making wise choices of goals with an individual, then ensuring proper preparation and allowing sensitive testing in small things. If the person attending has a disadvantage linked to their ability to learn, the centre involved in their care might be the first ever to enable a prize, a rosette or a pass grade to be gained.

For centres involved with teaching children, with or without physical disabilities or wider disadvantages, this approach will be very familiar and it is easily extrapolated to others of all ages.

Sometimes the individuals need to believe that they have the capacity to be successful and this is what needs to be enabled. This can be particularly true of people with a negative view of life for whatever reason. Self-confidence and self-belief are the characteristics that can enable people to try new things which may be necessary in therapy.

Again all centres could provide this intervention and those with more experienced and qualified teams will be providing it as part of a larger package as success is key for any activity. The provision does, however, require checks and balances to be in place. Producing false hope or inappropriate self-belief will be detrimental when the recipient is operating back in the real world and this must always be borne in mind.

A Level 1 centre would be following a plan written by someone else in which the goals will already have been set.

A Level 2 or 3 centre will be setting the goals and then providing the professional led intervention to ensure the good outcomes required for the recipient.

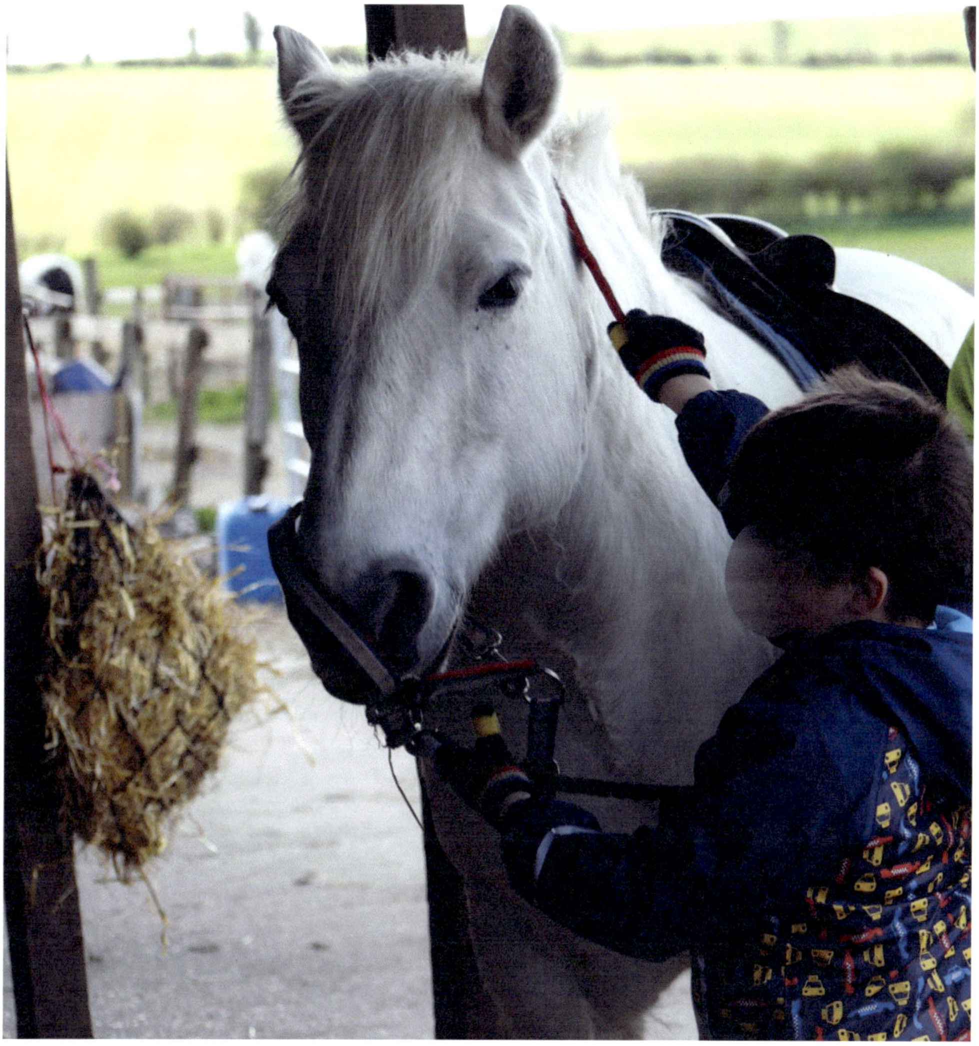

Image 9: A horse helping a human

Enabling success forms an excellent platform for all concentration work, mindfulness work or work based on grounding the over-excitable mind, for example in ADHD. The horse constantly calls the person back into the moment by their movement and reaction to the world. The cerebral stimulation of being outside and the emotional triggers from the horse help disordered brain patterns to be focused, giving much sought after clarity of thinking and concentration. This allows the team to enable the success for the person. This enhanced focus can at times be truly remarkable.

4.5.4 Self-awareness

Self-awareness is defined as being aware of one's own personality, feelings, strengths and weaknesses and thereby being able to interact with events, surroundings and others in a more effective way.

The therapeutic intervention to address this is the first which is fully Level 2 and would need to be led by a therapist with appropriate psychological skills. A therapy assistant can help to deliver a programme through prompting the recipient of the therapy but would need the oversight and supervision of the therapist.

Self-awareness can, of course, be taught anywhere but horses are particularly helpful in allowing the person to be truthful to themselves and others about the emotional aspect of their lives. Horses will show congruity between the feeling and the behaviour of the person engaged in the therapy. The learning from this can be used to assist the recipient to understand and then apply the learning to their own interactions with staff and others.

The first stages of learning to be self-aware involve discovering what personalities are, what feelings are and what effect behaviour has. This is then applied to the self with good and bad areas being noted. It may be that a cause for behaviour or unhelpful or heightened emotion is noticed and can be discussed.

During an assessment, or in the course of ongoing work, an area of difficulty such as poor concentration, leaving jobs unfinished, or talking over others is noticed and a decision is jointly made to change this area. The therapy assistant role would initially be to work alongside the recipient and remind them to finish a task, to use a coping strategy and so on, therefore reinforcing the possibility of change.

Experiences in life involving abusive relationships can cause people to lose self-awareness and consider themselves as invisible. For these people being noticed and accepted by a horse is hugely powerful, giving them a first step towards believing they can be noticed and accepted by others.

Once success is established doing activities on site the recipient can be encouraged to try certain things away from the centre. At their next visit they can learn more by discussing their self observation of the "off site" challenges with their therapist.

4.5.5 Education

One high level definition of education is described as a formative effect that arises from any experience. It can be seen that all centres teaching riding or ground based horse handling skills are educating their attendees.

In the outdoor therapy world education is usually meant as an alternative to mainstream education. As has already been described, young people with ADHD may be able to take in information whilst busy outside which they would not be able to absorb in a classroom environment.

It is clear that many life skills, knowledge, values of animal husbandry, good habits and team working are learned by the myriad of teenage girls who spend weekends and holidays helping at riding centres just for their own wellbeing.

What is being looked at here is the use of an outdoor setting, and a horse based one in particular, for the provision of education.

Education can be defined as facilitating learning and there are many people, young and old, who fall outside the normal distribution for learning (see reference to the normality in Chapter 1). This may be because of personal emotional difficulty, unusual learning styles, the inability to manage in large class sizes or other factors. Such people may be considered to have Special Educational Need or they may or may not have a statement of this need.

Schools and colleges in the UK have a requirement to provide education for their pupils and to seek alternative ways of teaching if the main classroom isn't suitable. Some of this extra provision will be given on site but this may not meet all needs. In these cases other educational provision should be sought. What the child or young person is trying to learn is usually stipulated by the school but it may be that the main curriculum of the country is not going to be practicable for an individual. A move to a vocational activity, taking up an apprenticeship or simply developing the ability to live more independently is what is needed instead.

A horse based establishment will have riding coaches on the staff. These people can provide knowledge and skills to the attendees and so facilitate learning. Centres working in partnership with local councils may be able to provide this and more, such as the Physical Education parts of a curriculum. Such work would be considered to be Level 1 as it is well within the ability of all properly appointed centres.

Local councils have further powers to define Providers of Alternative Education for the pupils in their county and the registration for this varies across county borders. Horse based centres are places where less formal educational settings are available and these may suit the learning styles of some students struggling in mainstream settings.

Forest School or Open Classroom sessions take place, teaching numeracy and literacy through field based activities at primary school level. This can be expanded to show science in action through observing biology, chemistry and physics around the daily activities of a yard. Whether weighing feeds, measuring height or weight of horses for worming programmes, discussing worm cycles or looking at soil PH the opportunities are endless. The geographical position of the centre and the description of its ground, map skills for outriding and the observation and understanding of weather add a whole further range of geography based possibilities that can be tailored to the individual student.

In addition to this there are transferable life skills, from horse care to personal care to consider. The need to rug a horse in winter can be used to teach about the need to dress appropriately for the weather at the yard. The need to shop for the horses' food, store and prepare it properly is transferred to learning about shopping for one's own meal, ensuring it is a well balanced diet, stored safely and eaten when fresh. The need for routine and time keeping, how to prepare for travel, what to do for minor illness and when and who to call for help, can all be taught well through transferable skills.

Curriculum based education can also work well in this environment but a centre providing full time education for 5 or more students of school age, whether or not the students have special educational needs, becomes considered a mainstream provider of education and under the governance of OFSTED. A qualified teacher working within a centre would not alone provide the cover needed to educate without registration as a school.

4.5.6 Communication

For humans and horses to work together there will need to be communication whether verbal, written or non-verbal. It is good to remember the old adage that communication is what is heard, or understood and not just what is said.

Communication at its simplest can be practised at a Level 1 centre but where there is recognised difficulty with this basic skill it would be better left to a centre with appropriately qualified staff.

Communication styles vary for all individuals and those with other disadvantages are no different. Some prefer loud, fast, expanded word counts and hyperbole whilst others, including those on the autistic spectrum prefer the complete opposite. People with disadvantages are also prone to all of the normal variation in communication skills and style as well as those connected to their disadvantage. For example, a young person with behavioural problems born out of an abusive past may have the difficulty of Attention deficit hyperactivity disorder (ADHD) and teenage challenge, in addition to the main concern of the awkward behaviour.

Amongst the complexity one thing is certain. In a therapeutic situation all communication needs to be appropriate, completely unambiguous and followed through. The latter may sound simple but is surprisingly difficult to manage within a team approach and poor communication and poor boundaries lie behind many an unhelpful behaviour.

In a normal therapeutic intervention the person engaged in therapy has only the therapist to communicate with. In outdoor therapy this is still the case. However, in horse based therapy a living animal is added to the session and one that doesn't simply respond to please them. Instead they need to communicate with it in order to take part in the activity.

The fact that the horse communicates non-verbally enables people to use this form of communication themselves and to read it where other people are concerned. When this has built their skill sufficiently words can be added in good time.

Learning to communicate better is something all people can benefit from, but for those with particular difficulty in communication any horse based activity will help.

4.5.7 Occupational therapy and physiotherapy

Occupational therapists and physiotherapists work in provision of treatments, rehabilitation and maintenance work. Occupational Therapy is a health science which seeks to develop, maintain or return people of all ages to a better level of function. This is done through identifying and eliminating barriers that prevent independence or participation in activities. Occupational therapists work with a holistic view of the person and would include all areas of disadvantage in their work whether physical, mental or behavioural.

These health professionals are goal orientated and these goals are shared between the therapist and their patient. In a horse-based setting the work includes adapting the environment, assisting the thinking, modifying tasks and helping with communication in order to allow participation and enable success. Skills learned at the centre can also help carers for the recipient of the therapy understand what is possible when at home and enable boundaries to be extended within the person's life.

Physiotherapy is a health science which uses specific exercises, manual treatments and manipulations, education and external devices to restore, improve or maintain movement and function. It is already widely practised outside the NHS in the UK with sports physiotherapists being perhaps the best known.

Physiotherapy is now becoming firmly established in outdoor therapy settings for rehabilitation and re-enablement and, in terms of horse-based work, the practice is widespread through organisations such as The Riding for the Disabled Association (RDA).

Physiotherapy aided by horses is such a growing interest for this professional group that they have a professional network, Association of Chartered Physiotherapists in Equine Activities (ACPEA), within their national body. This group describes itself as specialising in the use of the equine as a treatment modality.

The stated objectives of the group are to provide support and education to their members, promote high standards of practice and increase public and professional understanding of the work.

The work undertaken with horses can benefit people with functional disability of any origin whether from birth trauma, or after a stroke, or people seeking rehabilitation after an accident or operation or people with degenerative disease. All manner of horse-based activities are used to strengthen muscle groups and to improve range of movement of joints and aid recovery.

Groundwork can involve standing close to a horse and using it as an aid for balance. It could include grooming to increase range of movement through stretching or walking around a site. Individual programmes are easily compiled. For children the work in this area can prevent focus being on the disability, and receiving treatment, and rather on the fun aspect of the session in which therapy is surreptitiously delivered.

One significant therapeutic ability of the horse is that of moving the human body through the same three natural planes that are moved in human walking, as when the patient rides bare back under physiotherapist guidance. This area of work has been shown to provide remobilisation especially of the lower back beyond that of routine, plinth-based physiotherapy treatments. This is because bareback riding facilitates movement in all three planes of rotation, essentially a "3D workout" takes place.

During normal walking, a healthy human pelvis, lower spine and hips all move freely in three planes of orientation of pitch, roll and yaw. Pitch is the movement required to bend a person over to touch their toes. Roll is the movement which allows the sliding of a hand down the outer edge of a leg to the knee. Yaw is the movement of rotating the front of the pelvis to point left or right of straight ahead. As the spine is one linked structure, the movement at the lower spine also produces movement in the thoracic and cervical spine at the same time, which is why such interventions need oversight of experienced physiotherapists.

Both Occupational therapists and Physiotherapists have professional groups who meet to share knowledge and standards of working in the field of Outdoor Therapy and particularly in the area of Equine Assisted Therapies.

4.5.8 Psychological therapies

In Chapter 1, I explained the view that therapeutic interventions used in the outdoors should be those which are already nationally accepted. This is logical and reasonable as there are a wide range of therapeutic interventions already in existence.

This range is supported by established toolkits for interventions and monitoring of progress through accredited questionnaires and recording processes. In order for a service to provide psychological therapy to Level 2 it needs to have an appropriately qualified member of the team who has adequate supervision and governance for independent practice.

For people considering equine or horse-based psychological therapy an understanding of the type of intervention that is being offered by the therapist at a centre is sensible and so the following overview of that which is currently available within the UK is given. Whilst all are effective some may feel more accessible than others in terms of style of delivery.

The therapies can be roughly categorised as:-

- those effecting behaviour change, e.g Cognitive Behavioural Therapy (CBT)
- the psychoanalytical and psychodynamic which look for relationship patterns unconsciously developed in childhood
- the humanistic therapies which look for self-awareness and change in the present
- art and play therapies
- other therapies with national recognition now include the Eye Movement Desensitisation and Reprogramming (EMDR) treatment used to aid emotional processing in trauma resolution

- family therapy
- mindfulness

but clearly there are many more.

Many therapists have a special interest in one area of work initially but then adopt others and so enlarge the range of interventions that they can offer people.

Family therapy is well delivered by ground based work with horses as are relationship issues in general.

The cognitive and behavioural therapy group offers several categories. These include behavioural therapy, cognitive therapy, combined CBT, Acceptance and Commitment Therapy (ACT) and Cognitive and Analytic therapy (CAT).

The Humanistic Group has even more to offer within the envelope of person-centred work with options such as Solution Focussed Brief Intervention Therapy and Human Givens Psychotherapy.

Art Therapy and Drama Therapy are easily integrated into outdoor practice as the recording of the feelings engendered by the outside and the horse lead to creativity expressed through art. When guided and explored with a therapist the art exposes internal emotions which can be addressed. The use of drama to enact being bullied or practise the avoidance of bullying using horses and boundaries is both powerful and very effective.

Each of these therapies relies on an array of tools used in therapeutic interactions with recipients. The purpose of the book is only to assist those who are unfamiliar with this field to understand what is available, rather than give an exhaustive list which those in the field recognise.

Such tools may also include thought diaries in some format, it may include personality profiling, consideration of thinking styles and looking for causes for current problems in the past.

In considering psychological therapy it is essential that no recipient should have two parallel treatment programmes running. One will certainly interfere with the other and any centre providing psychological intervention must be clear who is holding responsibility for the case. If responsibility is held by a mainstream service provider the centre should work to the plan and offer general support to this but avoid any new therapeutic intervention unless in discussion with the lead therapist.

Whilst an intervention as apparently straightforward as active listening may be of great value and could be provided by a therapy assistant, it can only be provided with appropriate training and close supervision from a qualified therapist.

The psychological aspects of the Certificate In Equine Coaching (CIEC) level 2 coaching awards do give some basic training in how people think and how to assist individuals to improve-but this should not be confused with a therapeutic intervention.

4.5.9 Conditions that are able to benefit from horse related therapy

The following is a list of conditions in no particular order which are already known to be assisted by horse-based work:-

- work related stress
- life events and adjustment disorders
- anxiety and depression
- social anxiety
- school refusal
- challenging behaviour
- Obsessive Compulsive Disorder (OCD)
- Personality Disorder and traits
- Attention Deficit Hyperactivity Disorder (ADHD)
- adoption or rejection issues
- Post Traumatic Stress Disorder (PTSD)
- bullying
- childhood attachment issues
- domestic violence
- self-harm in young people
- physical injury
- post operative recovery
- rehabilitation
- Chronic Fatigue Syndrome
- bereavement
- substance misuse
- low self-confidence
- abusive relationship sequelae
- trauma, both physical and mental

- learning difficulties
- anger management
- Autistic Spectrum Disorder (ASD)

4.6 Horse-based areas of application

The attention of this book now changes to the other axis of the horse-based therapy matrix to give an understanding of the applications themselves and the therapeutic interventions in which they can be used. See Fig. 15 earlier in this chapter.

The importance of each activity is not shown on the generic horse-based matrix. For this to be shown a further matrix would be needed, one which expanded the possibilities of an activity along the x axis by removing all other activities as shown below.

Each area of application, or horse-based activity, will be used for therapeutic benefit and the rules of application are not similar across all the activities on the matrix. Bareback riding

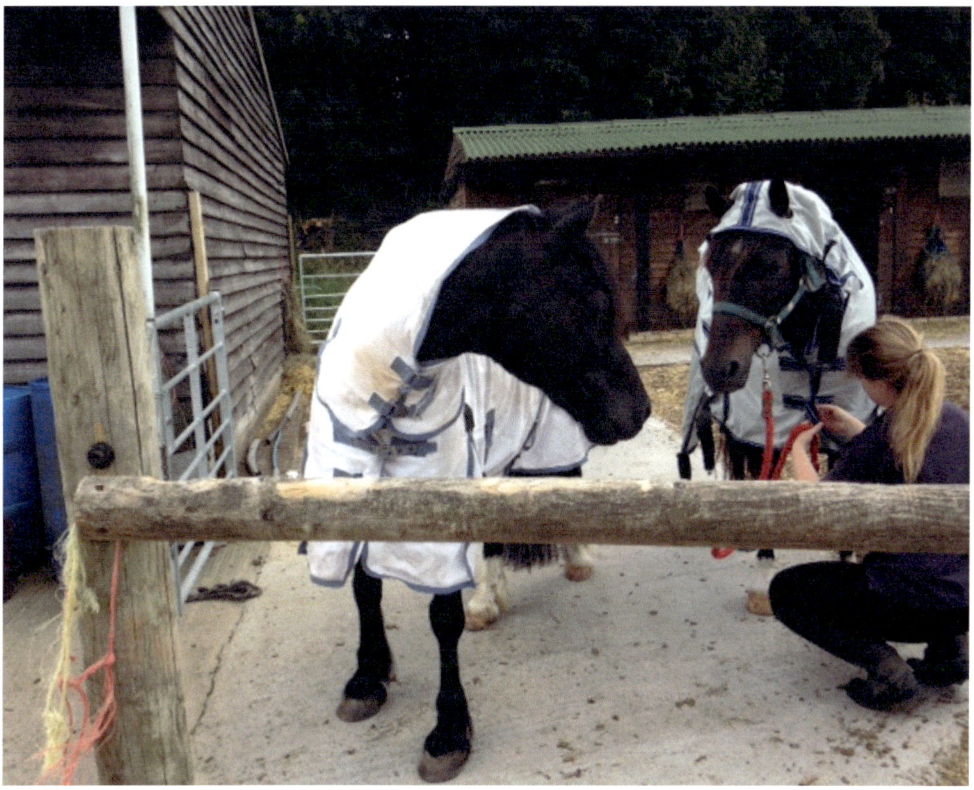

Image 10: Helping with the flies

is likely only to be practised for half an hour whilst field management could be accessed all day. Bareback riding could not be practised alone but safe field management could be.

4.6.1 Field management

This wonderful and unending area of activity gives limitless seasonal, agricultural and self-awareness activities. People can be enabled to succeed in finding ragwort, horse poo collecting, fencing repairs, etc. They can be taught to notice the effect of the weather and the seasons upon grazing and equine behaviour. They can take part in team working or learn to work for extending periods of time on their own. If the main yard is busy they can go to a paddock for some peaceful time and can have all manner of jobs created for them to provide purposeful activity whilst out in the field.

Most teams within the horse world see this as a less important area and certainly not as a therapeutic one. Exercising horses is perceived as more fun by most, and teaching the importance of less exciting jobs is a life skill that deserves attention.

All centres can provide this activity which works with all eight therapeutic areas.

4.6.2 Bareback riding

Bareback riding does not mean allowing riders free rein to gallop without saddles. It is an activity designed to:-

- further relaxation
- allow those with less than perfect childhoods to be carried
- allow those who feel powerless to be in communion with a powerful animal
- train people in mindfulness
- build core strength and balance
- encourage silence for a while

Bareback riding in therapy is not about riding but about being led. It is done with a back pad or a completely bare saddle area and always with a leader.

If the bareback riding is for someone engaged in a low back pain therapy they simply sit astride, they do not ride. This is a fully led session where the horse's leader is not providing therapy but provides the safety for the whole team, i.e. the recipient, the horse, the therapist and themselves. This leaves the therapist free to watch the movement produced and suggest movement and exercises as appropriate.

If a physiotherapy led session is to improve core stability or muscle tone the session may well take place with a non slip back pad instead of a saddle. Back pads are usually less likely to be used for riders with poor balance but they are a better option as the heat from direct contact with the horses back increases the effectiveness of the therapy. Competent side-walkers are therefore essential to prevent sideways slipping of the rider.

If the bareback session is being used for psychological therapy the heat of direct contact is again beneficial. In this case a back pad to aid balance is preferable to two side walkers being added to the team as they may add distractions. Riding bare back, being led and carried, can be emotionally powerful and the deeply hidden emotions which may surface are better managed with a smaller team.

Bareback riding can be used across therapeutic interventions 1, 3, 4, 7 and 8 but could be used across all as part of an individual programme if a therapist is available.

4.6.3 Back riding

Back riding is the technique of a trained rider sitting behind the person engaged in therapy while mounted and moving upon the horse. This again has many therapeutic possibilities but the combined weight of the human load must be within the carrying weight range of the horse. Horse movement brings constant movement to the human body when riding whether bareback or saddled. The use of a saddle minimises this movement which is likely to be preferable unless a therapist has specifically designed the session to be bareback.

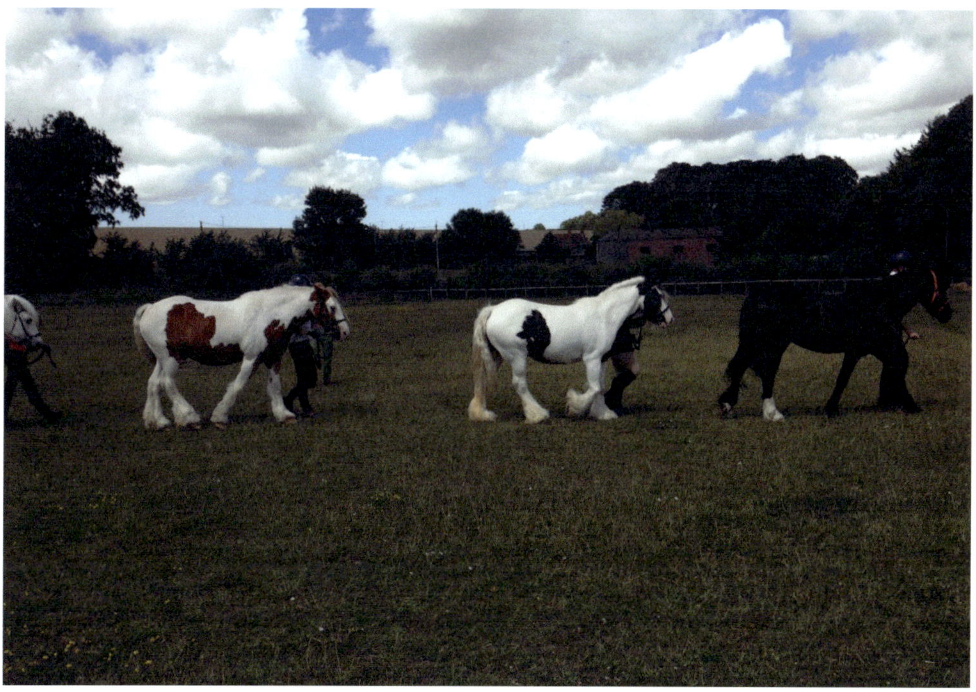

Image 11: Learning to show in hand

Back riding can produce a great feeling of freedom for someone unable to sit unaided in the saddle and has been used to gradually improve core stability to such a level that the rider can then ride alone.

This technique was widely publicised by Rupert Isaacson in The Horse Boy and is available at several centres throughout the UK.

Back riding is always a useful part of a therapeutic programme, it can enable all kinds of goals to be reached including simply having fun.

4.6.4 Competition

The ability to compete in life is an essential skill for resilient living whether it is to access a share in an essential commodity, voice personal wishes or dislikes on simple matters or, at the other end of the spectrum, learning to lose graciously.

Centres can enable all the work around competition, including preparation and planning, managing nervousness and keeping perspective. The aim may be to transfer such skills to other areas of life such as attending school, not being bullied and taking exams successfully.

Competition is particularly useful in areas 3 to 8 of the therapeutic interventions.

4.6.5 Driving

Centres that can offer driving have a whole new set of skills to offer both the able-bodied and the disadvantaged. This form of equine activity can lead to partnership with a horse, working with the team, competition and the need for equine care just as in other activities but has new equipment, language and skills to add.

Wheelchair driving can allow the special feeling of freedom to a wheelchair user who would not be able to ride, moving cross country (or field!) by driving the horse themselves or with an able-bodied whip.

Communication amongst team members, spatial awareness and personal stability are all needed for driving and the capacity to enable success and self-confidence are self evident. Rehabilitation may mean freedom for a previously fit person who now becomes a wheelchair whip or for someone with mental health problems who learns to groom for an able-bodied person and combat fear, experience belonging and exhilaration. Driving can be used across all 8 areas of therapeutic interventions.

4.6.6 Ethogram work

This is the study of the horse in its natural habitat and in a herd. Clearly when done in a field this only gives part of the picture but aspects of the behaviour can be observed when animals are turned out regularly into a large paddock in the same group.

Hierarchy, interactions and movements that convey meanings can all be seen and the observer needs to use patience and stillness together with observational skills and writing.

This area of work is useful when encouraging self-directed learning. The horses themselves act as the prompts without the need to be prompted by a facilitator. Whatever the goal of the therapy the ethogram work is good for lengthening periods of quiet, of stillness, or reduced stimulation for those on the Autistic Spectrum. Ethograms act as a conduit for learning transferrable skills in making sense of the world and understanding behaviour of people.

Ethogram work can be useful in mental illness including Post Traumatic Stress Disorder as it can be used to relearn the skill of looking at surroundings without the heightened perception of threat which often challenges military veterans in many therapy settings.

Ethogram work can be used in therapeutic interventions 3-8 although in an individual programme the application may have uses in therapeutic interventions 1 and 2.

4.6.7 Groundwork

Groundwork in this setting means leading or working with the horse often at liberty in an arena. It is a strong component of psychological and behavioural work with horses. Much horse based therapy takes place unmounted which means that riding weight isn't an issue, nor is horse size nor behaviour under saddle, so increasing the opportunities for people to access the work.

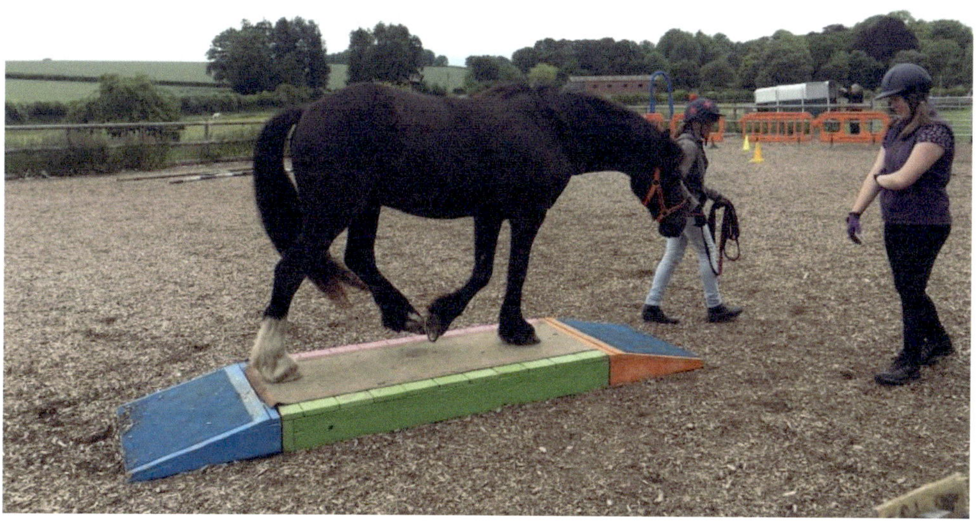

Image 12: Ground based agility work

Ground work is again a very wide application and can take place in groups, including family groups, as well as one to one. Horses can be attached by a long line or loose in the field or arena and much can be taught and demonstrated using this application. It teaches people about themselves, their communication style, their assertiveness and about relationships within their family. The therapeutic interventions seem less personal and threatening when delivered outside and using a horse to help demonstrate. Non-verbal communication, planning and perseverance are all exercised in this work.

In chemistry, a catalyst makes the chemical reaction proceed much more swiftly and the horse is sometimes described as a catalyst for this reason. The value of using a horse can be very powerful in the acceleration of understanding and change.

4.6.8 Horse agility

Horse Agility is a growing aspect of horse competition and is ground based and suited to all. It can teach humans to communicate differently with different horses, to take on new challenges, to compete locally or even on-line using videoed performance and to work towards personal goals.

4.6.9 Horsecare

Horse care is an activity which appeals to some potential recipients hence its inclusion in the list. This is the gentle side of animal husbandry and is a good name for those who don't yet see that stable management is really the same thing. Horsecare can include all aspects of horse welfare including field management, daily routine, overseeing exercise or feeding and grooming. Rugging, care of rugs and tack, and mucking out all contribute to care of the horse, which is why stable management would cover this work too, but horse care can allow time to simply "be" in the horses presence. Horsecare works strongly in therapeutic intervention areas 1 and 2. It is very affirming to see a horse react to the recipient's arrival at feeding time. Using horsecare to teach boundaries and responsibilities such as " no one leaves until the horses are comfortable" is widely used in residential care in the USA for behaviourally disturbed young people and adults with substance misuse problems.

Horsecare has a role within all 8 therapeutic interventions on the matrix.

4.6.10 Connection

Connection centres on the communication that the horse uses and how people can learn to understand this in order to better connect to the equine. Although established to help horses and save handers time it has since been recognised to provide significant psychological benefit to the handler, including military veterans with PTSD.

4.6.11 Longlining

Longlining is an equine ground based activity in its own right and not just a training aid for a young horse or something offered by those who don't have a carriage for driving.

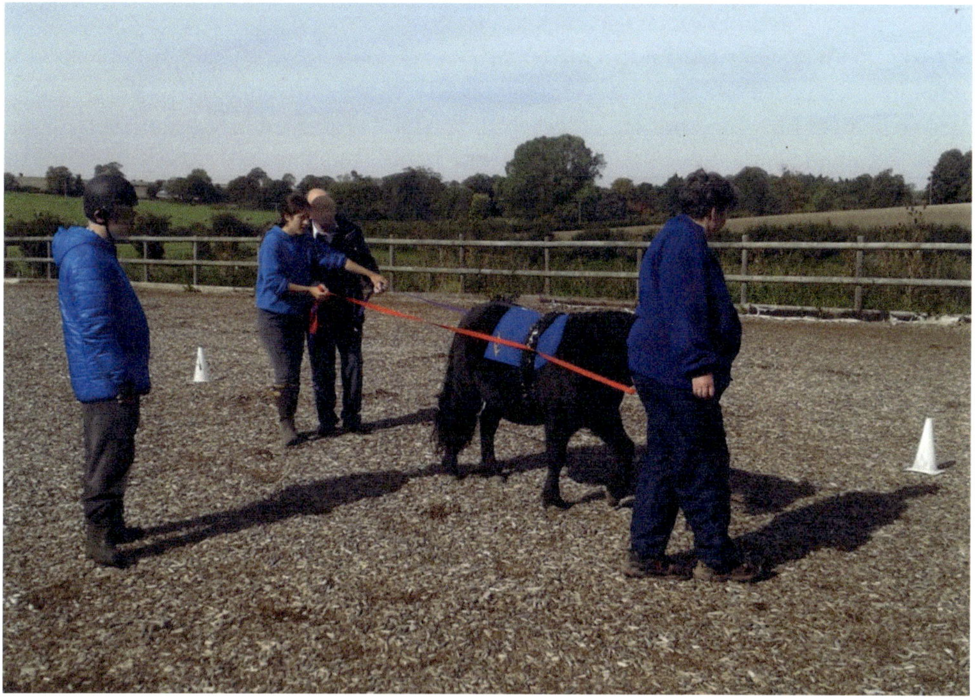

Image 13: Longlining for therapy

Longlining requires physical fitness but can also be used with wheelchair users. It requires concentration, communication and learning of skills in order to follow a course. Like any area of work with horses some self-assertiveness is useful and as this is exerted at a greater distance it will need to be more strongly exercised. The use of different coloured lines helps with recognition of right and left and the intervention can be done silently which is often useful for those with Autistic Spectrum Disorder (ASD) and others with communication difficulties.

Longlining is mainly useful in areas 1 and 3, 4, 5, 7 and 8 although an individual programme may find application in 2 and 6.

4.6.12 Riding as a sport

The benefits of horse riding as a sport are evident to many who will read this book. People enjoy horse riding and this is effectively another tool to be considered as potential therapy. The benefits include:-

- improved physical fitness
- improved mood from being outside
- improved mood from relationships with horse and others
- improved mood from feeling included in a hobby that can be talked about
- being enabled to succeed

Moving this on through simple tests such as the Association of British Riding Schools (ABRS) weekly rider test series gives riders the opportunity of learning about their own response to stressful situations in life and how they might manage their stress better. Tests or exams do not need to be high level but are an excellent way of learning concentration, preparation, team work and aiding growth in self-confidence as the recipient understands what constitutes success.

Clearly the testing available is defined by whatever system the riding centre or its coach or instructor uses to show improvement in riding skill as a sport. This area of activity can be used to cover the first 5 areas of therapeutic intervention on the matrix.

Once "riding with goals" has produced sufficient improvement it is often a natural progression to return to learning in the mainstream setting. This will help to achieve a main aim of rehabilitation.

4.6.13 Riding with goals

Riding with goals is particularly useful for someone who is unable to manage mainstream lessons as part of their therapy. This inability may be due to their being too driven, too fearful, too shy or less able to concentration or communicate. Riding with goals doesn't need to be a 1 to 1 session it can still be a group session in which each rider follows their own route to successful completion of their individual goals. Such sessions may or may not include the actual learning of riding as a sport but may be concerned with other learning, for example being able to ride for longer, learning to concentrate, sitting up without assistance, manage very basic control of the horse or perhaps being silent on the horse's back whilst trying to hear what else is going on.

A ridden activity such as this can be a useful way of working toward the same goals as are being worked on during a half day visit. Working on concentration or using the right hand more fully whilst in field management, then in horse care and then in riding with goals, reinforces the message each time the activity is changed. The overall outcome of the half day can be improved for certain recipients through the changes, rather than using one activity for the whole visit. Riding with goals can be used across all 8 therapeutic Intervention areas.

4.6.14 Stable management

Some centres will offer this activity and testing for it as part of their preferred system of showing progress. This area of activity can be used to cover all 8 areas of therapeutic intervention on the matrix and can lead on towards vocational qualifications if so wished. The teaching of stable management is a mainstream subject in the equine industry and in a therapeutic setting it is often a natural progression after Horse Care.

4.6.15 Training the horse

Training the horse is an activity with as many applications as field management. All horses need occasional reminders about what is acceptable, especially those in busy riding centres where the handling they receive is not always consistent. Horses also benefit from doing something different occasionally, perhaps learning about a new ground based challenge, and involving someone receiving therapy in this work can be very valuable. Training a horse often needs a second person to assist and this alone could be used with therapeutic interventions 1-6. The balance for any such session can be changed from the trainer having their attention on the horse to the trainer acting in a therapeutic role with the human keeping the horse safe. Any horse, no matter how much in need of training, will act as a therapist for the human by demonstrating how behaviour has an effect, how emotions affect others and what resisting change can look like. Certain horses can also be useful to show a young and over confident male that perhaps they still have things to learn.

Working with young horses can be really useful in assisting adults with emotional, mental and behavioural problems. Clearly young horses are less predictable and less forgiving of human misjudgement or miscommunication so programmes such as this should be considered Level 3 only. Young horses can be adversely affected by poor or inconsistent handling and may not cope well with high emotional load. Furthermore they represent the opposite of a good therapy horse as they will be inconsistent and the handler cannot predict their reactions. Such programmes always need to be closely supervised by a competent horse person.

Rehabilitation programmes for horses are now starting to offer targeted work for humans. Many barns in the USA only work with horses needing rehabilitation. This provides a similar range of behaviours to manage as working with youngstock although in rehabilitation the unhelpful horse behaviour will be established. Such programmes in the USA continue to gain funding because of the benefit they bring to both horse and human.

4.6.16 Vaulting

Vaulting is a recognised activity performed with a horse on a lunge line. The able bodied aspect of the sport is described as dance or gymnastics on the back of the moving horse. It can be undertaken in a group setting or with only the support of the horse and the experienced handler. In this activity a well balanced and well trained horse who can trot or canter at a consistent pace around a 15 metre circle whilst being lunged is used. Such a horse will need to have the capacity to carry weight and vaulting should only be taught by those with appropriate qualifications in this field.

Vaulting can be used within the therapeutic setting by using simple exercises in walk or possibly trot. It can be used in all 8 therapeutic areas.

4.6.17 Volunteering

Most centres could successfully offer volunteering to those who are interested. Centres need to be aware, however, that not all volunteers are equally able. The mark of a useful volunteer is someone who adds to the overall provision, taking less time being supervised than they give back through work done. Then this is a genuine offer of free help to the organisation. Many who offer to volunteer are really those who need a supported placement and a centre must recognise and understand how to handle this. The amount of supervision that a volunteer requires to be safe determines the level of staff support that will need to be available during the visit. The amount of supervision required helps the team understand whether this needs to attract funding to cover staff costs or is indeed a genuine offer of free help for the organisation.

Managing volunteers, no matter how committed, is a challenge for all organisations and takes more time than may be expected. Induction needs to be undertaken and the need for confidentiality for those attending for therapy explained and required. Clarity about what a volunteer would like to be involved in, and being assessed for their ability to undertake this, should take place before any agreement is reached to avoid disappointment on either or both sides later on.

A commercial yard may be less keen to offer supported volunteering placements whilst a charitable therapy yard could use this across all 8 therapeutic interventions.

4.6.18 Wheelchair work

Wheelchair work is the term applied for activities across the whole range that can be offered to someone in a wheelchair. A wheelchair user can be enabled to take part in field management, back riding, bareback riding, riding as a sport or with goals, and all manner of ground based activities including longlining. Activity undertaken will be selected for the level of their ability with due regard to safety and their disadvantage. Working with youngstock or training of horses would seem to be unwise for most using a wheelchair due to the need to move quickly at times and the lower level of the wheelchair beside the animal.

What is needed to allow wheelchair working is adequate staffing, sufficient understanding of wheelchair constraints and adequate ease of access to good surfaces and well trained horses. This is definitely an area in which a horse needs to have received specific training and shown themselves consistently suited to the work. Wheelchair work when available can deliver across all 8 therapeutic interventions

4.6.19 Work experience

A centre should interpret requests for work experience as a sign of acceptance within its local community. The extra work, including that of supervising the student, should be accepted whenever possible as a positive return for good, local relationships. Young people seeking work experience in a therapeutic setting need to be carefully supervised in terms of the confidentiality that those attending for therapy are entitled to and are better employed only under the heading of Groom Assistant. A young person with a disadvantage may also apply for work experience so that they are able to experience what a working day is like even though they would be unable to access this experience elsewhere. Such a young person may well need considerable supervision and therefore the centre may need to access funding or bursary funds for such a placement.

Providing work experience for a young person with disadvantage would cover the first 5 areas of therapeutic intervention and so would be a valuable step in the young person's life. The purpose of the placement will be outlined by the referring education provider and is an opportunity to approach time keeping, work rate, resilience and team working across the groom based activities. Unless a special arrangement is made it would not be expected for a young person to be riding during the placement unless already an accomplished rider.

Work experience placements may also be requested for college students and university students. Such placements may be in general horse care for roles in the equine industry or for emerging roles of therapeutic application such as physiotherapy or occupational therapy. Once again the centre should be clear that the extra pair of hands may not actually add much to the completion of the daily work but that teaching others about the work, answering questions and observing the excitement at progress made by recipients is good for the well-being of the centre's team.

4.7 Endless possibilities

Each area of the matrix has now been considered and the levels of therapeutic complexity within which teams can safely operate have been explored.

If a centre wished to specialise in just one area the matrix will still work well as a means of visually explaining the centre's provision to a potential funder or recipient.

In the simple mathematical diagram at fig.16 sub categories have been added showing the increasing possibilities. Each letter on the x axis could be matched with each number on the y axis giving 16 possibilities per box. This is clearly too complex to work with sensibly when each option in a therapy matrix is described by words.

Fig. 16: Mathematical possibilities matrix

	A, A.1,A.2,A.3	B,B1,B2,B3	C,C1,C2,C3
1 1.1 1.2 1.3			
2 2.1 2.2 2.3		2B 2.1B 2.3B2	
3 3.1 3.2 3.3			

Education Matrix

Name:	Tutor/coach:	Date:

Level	Considerations	Areas of Application																				
Prov Alt Ed	Age Disadvantage and Severity 1:1 or group	Agriculture	Abseiling	Climbing	Cycling	Camping	Countryside Skills	Canoe and Kayaking	Ecology	Exped and Adventure	Forestry	Horticulture	Horse Based activity	Nav and Orienteering	Running	Sailing and Windsurfing	Surfing	Walking	Wilderness	Volunteering	Work Experience	OTHER
Education offered		**Possibilities available**																				
Basic numeracy																						
Basic literacy																						
Concept of humanities																						
Concept of race and language																						
Basic science																						
IT																						
Problem solving																						
PE																						
Life Skills																						

Fig. 17: Example of education matrix in use at a Level 3 Outdoor Therapy Centre

If each area of therapeutic intervention is taken and expanded with its subcategories a different range of possibilities arises. In Fig. 17. the area of Education has been expanded to show its components and this is used as an example with the outcome that all the possibilities across the Areas of Application now have an education focus.

Any centre wishing to provide horse based therapy could define and create its own Offer Matrix and the possibilities are, indeed, endless.

Case Study 4

Jackie was a 36 year old local lady who had been to an Open Day at the centre. She had attended the event with a friend whose children came to Gul. Jackie had brought her own children to the Open Day and all had enjoyed it. She had seen the demonstration on back pain. She made enquiries to come and meet a physiotherapist at the yard to discuss her own pain.

When aged 17 years old Jackie had been involved in a road traffic accident in which the vehicle she was travelling in was hit from behind and she suffered a form of whiplash as a consequence. She described a period of headaches while going through college and much of this discomfort was put down to the stress of academic work rather than to the whiplash though this probably had contributed.

During both of her pregnancies she suffered considerable low back pain, mostly arising from the sacroiliac joints, but when the second child was nine months she picked him up awkwardly producing an episode of sciatica. This settled but four years later, on returning to work as an administrative assistant for the MOD, she started spending large periods of time sitting at a computer desk. This caused a recurrence of discomfort sufficient to require time off work. The Occupational Health Department and the GP worked well to mitigate her discomfort and Jackie was able to work again but had regular discomfort which often disrupted her sleep over the following four years.

Jackie, on presentation, was clearly low in mood. She was contending with working 28 hours per week, managing a home with two fairly active boys in it who needed full time care when not in school and had been promoted at work which added to workplace stress levels. Her interrupted sleep was not helping.

On her assessment forms Jackie had given permission for Gul to discuss her case with her GP if that should be necessary. The senior physiotherapist took a careful history and then examined the range of movements in Jackie's back. She was clearly very stiff in the lumbosacral region and had areas of facet joint tenderness in the mid-thoracic spine.

Hip adduction was good with a full range of movement in the hips and there was no current sciatic nerve involvement.

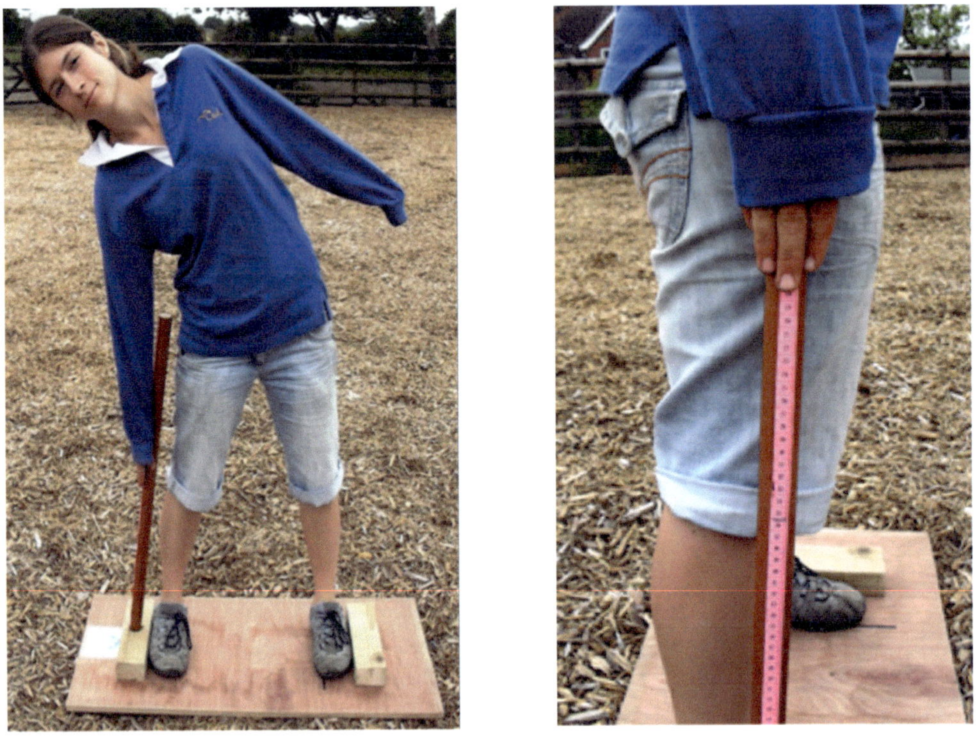

Image 14: Side flexion measurement demonstrated by a staff member

A trial of bare back riding therapy was agreed and Jackie was sent away with rider forms to complete prior to her return at a suitable and mutually convenient time.

The physiotherapist was very well aware of the stresses already working in Jackie's life and, knowing the power of the equine work, knew that this needed to be approached very gently to avoid precipitating more discomfort by too robust an approach.

On Jackie's arrival at the yard for her first session her lateral flexion was measured as an indicator for mobility and the analogue scale of pain taken.

The physiotherapist discussed the programme with Jackie. This was riding bareback at the walk with one side walker in a straight line with one large turn and return. The intention was that this first episode should take no more than 10 minutes and an assessment of pain levels immediately afterwards, one day afterwards and two days afterwards would be taken. Jackie agreed to the careful recording of symptoms at home after the session had taken place.

The horse chosen for this session was a 14 hand solidly built cob mare, Josie. Josie's long eyelashes, long mane and gentle nature appeals to most ladies, particularly those with low mood.

Jackie was mounted carefully from the mounting block using the side mount with 3 members of staff to ensure a safe and painless mount for this first session.

The movement of the mare, Josie, is fairly flat and slow thereby producing a gentle introduction to mobilising the lower spine. At the end of the ride, Jackie's mood had lifted as she had really enjoyed the session. She was already looking forward to returning to ride Josie bareback in the coming weeks. The side flexion was checked and had improved by 2cm on the right and 3cm on the left, Jackie was thrilled. There was no pain during the session and none immediately afterwards.

Jackie recorded a good night sleep on the first night but some increased stiffness on the following two days which then settled. A full programme was confirmed with Jackie on her return the following week.

During the course of the next 6 weeks the physiotherapist noticed the right side was less flexible than the left and so, still using Josie, circles were walked on the left rein in walk causing an increased right side stretch. Clearly the number of straight lines and circles is managed by the physiotherapist to avoid overworking the area of the spine that is being stretched.

Jackie reported diminished pain, improved mood, better sleep and enjoying her family more. An interesting side element to this therapeutic intervention, and exactly the sort of thing that happens when using horses, was the disclosure that Jackie had always wished for a girl child but her two children were both boys. This need to mother in a different way was a sadness for her that had contributed to tension and reaction and mood. She found grooming Josie and being carried by the horse an opportunity to come to terms with her motherhood and felt better for this.

One year on, Jackie does not attend regularly but phones approximately every three or four months to book for three or four sessions to "mobilise" her back and chat through her current life issues.

Chapter 5

Selection, training and care of horses for therapy

5.0 Selection of therapy horses

Horses are selected for use in therapy in two ways, firstly through a loan agreement or purchase, and secondly through deciding which horse is most suitable for a session from the horses available at the centre.

In order to successfully select a horse for therapy it is key to know the role it is to fulfil.

In the case of a centre with an established provision and a selection of horses already available, the purpose of the new purchase or loan may be to fill the one size, shape, skill or behaviour that the centre doesn't otherwise have. Alternatively it may be to provide another steady weight-carrier to share the load of the other horses currently doing this work.

Whilst a role can be established for most horses it is wiser to have a role identified before agreeing to a loan or purchase and the centre's own offer matrix will assist in this.

In my practice I have found that the only essential characteristic of the therapy horse is consistency. The animal needs to be consistently quiet or consistently challenging, consistently reflective and so on. All other characteristics can be worked with, whatever the horse's history and personality, but consistency is key.

If the horse is to be used only for groundwork its size and behaviour under saddle, and to some extent its conformation, become less important. If, however, it is to be used for physical therapy and bareback riding it needs to be solidly built, preferably with "a leg at each corner", calm in nature and up to weight but not too tall. If the horse is over 14 hands 2inches high it is considerably more difficult for the therapy team to assist with complex mounting or dismounting, or managing poor balance with a rider.

5.1 Characteristics of therapy horses

The characteristic of a good temperament means a calm and non-confrontational animal. Such an animal represents a good choice for any therapy as they are likely to allow people to move around them in stables, yards and fields without undue concern. Whilst people attending therapy yards, whether disadvantaged or not, are advised on safe practice around horses, such as not going under the belly of the animal, they are on average less able and less likely to follow the advice.

Care should be taken over the animal's health and conformation as a poor choice can leave the centre with unwanted and potentially avoidable veterinary and farriery costs.

More centres providing ground based work and therapy are now considering barefoot (unshod) management of horses if the road work is light enough. The benefits of this are considerable. The barefoot horse means less injury to trodden on human feet, less concern within herd groups and better shock absorption and balance for horses who carry unbalanced loads.

The health of an animal for loan or purchase needs to be fully explored in order to avoid unwanted surprises such as seasonal conditions or intermittent lameness. Less than perfect health is not a barrier to acquisition as no animal will be perfect and the management of health conditions can be used in an educational manner for those attending. Excessive health needs, however, would add costs, take time and detract from the centre's overall ability to provide.

In addition to knowing the horse's health its life history should be looked into if possible, as its experiences and behaviour in various settings could affect which roles it will be able to undertake in therapy.

The gender of a horse will affect its behaviour and there are three genders to consider; stallion, mare and gelding. The gender of a new horse can be an issue for horse management at a centre. Mares are more variable in moods due to hormonal cycles but can also be more perceptive and intuitive than geldings. Their role in the herd can be to lead, to manage the unruly behaviour of growing foals and yearlings and, of course, to suckle and raise young. A mare that has foaled is often aware of pregnancy in humans and is usually interested in small children. A mare may also be more tolerant of annoying behaviour in humans with learning disabilities showing their ability to differentiate. They have the capacity to soak up more emotion but can also be quite challenging if they have a lead mare personality.

Geldings are believed to make good riding horses because their behaviour remains consistent with no concern over spring time behaviour, however those who were gelded late may still exhibit some unwelcome stallion like tendencies within the herd.

Stallions are far less likely to be used in therapy but a well trained stallion can certainly be an asset to a centre.

5.2 Training for therapy

The training of a horse for therapy is essentially no different to training a horse for any other activity. Horses learn at different rates and some can learn more complex procedures and commands more quickly than others. In all horse training the task to be learned needs to be broken down and the horse allowed to learn it stage by stage. Horses learn with repetition and will need to have refresher training if they are to manage something calmly when they haven't done it for some time.

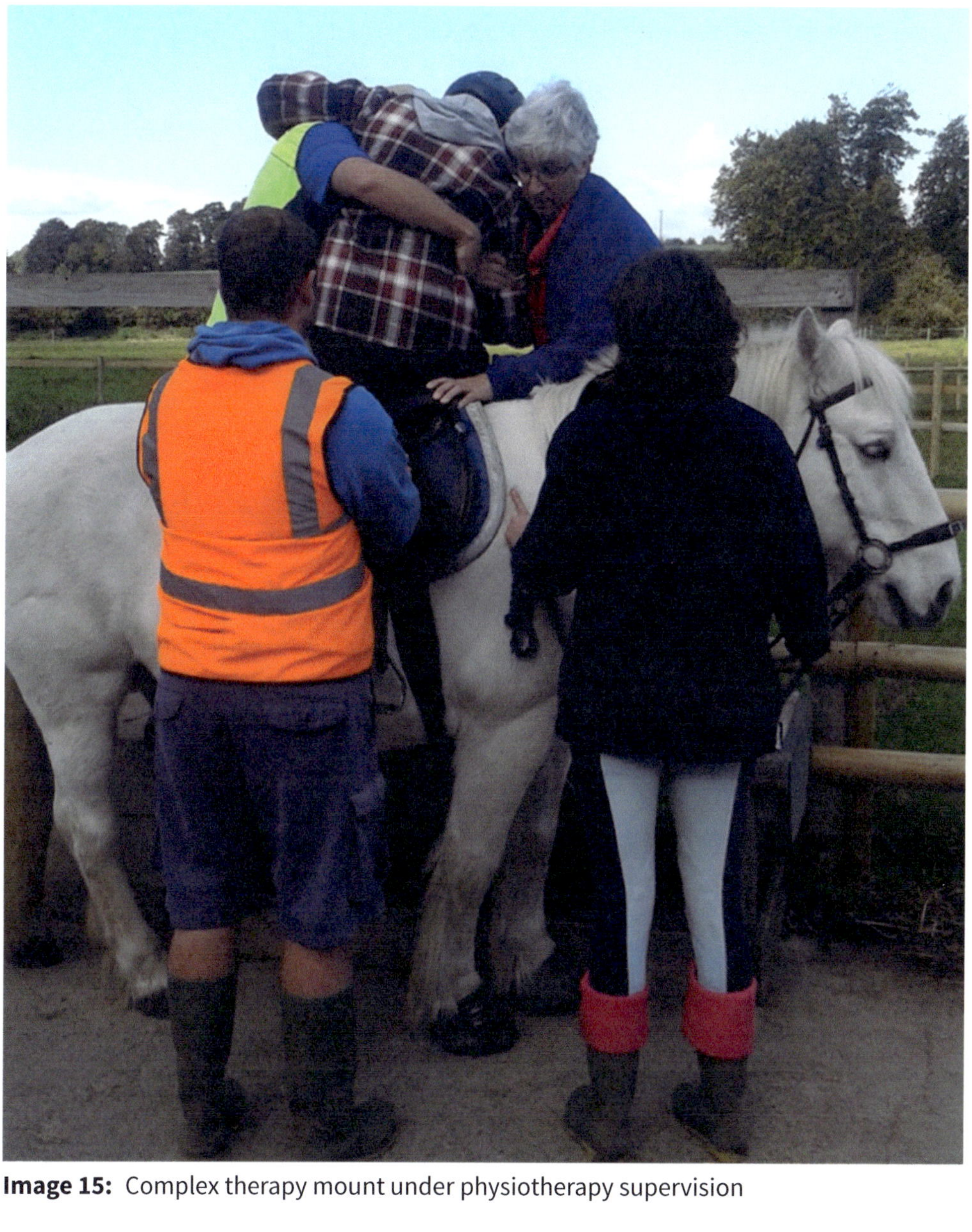

Image 15: Complex therapy mount under physiotherapy supervision

A complex mount for a disadvantaged person may be undertaken pelvis first and with the person sitting sideways on the saddle from the mounting block as the first step. Such a mount can take as many as 5 assistants around the horse and the horse needs to be trained to expect this and know what will happen next. The full sequence of events is outlined below:-

- walk up straight to the mounting block
- halt square
- move individual legs on command to adjust position
- be comfortable with the mounting block very close
- stand still until told to move
- tolerate people all around, phase 1 training is to start with 5 people on the ground only and progress to then working with two people on the block and others on the ground for a normal mount with many assistants
- complex mount with the rider being lowered pelvis first to sit sideways on the saddle
- lower head on command
- allow leg to pass over their head whilst assistants are very close
- allow repositioning of the rider which can take some time
- brace for and accommodate the oddly balanced load
- move away and walk with many people around

5.2.1 Wheelchair training

For a horse to work successfully with a wheelchair user it needs to have training. This is easily undertaken using able bodied staff and chairs. A horse used in this area needs to learn to approach the wheelchair from a side angle initially.

The horse needs to learn to stand steadily with a wheelchair close to its shoulder, flank or quarters to allow grooming. Horses should be taught to walk quietly with their able bodied handler on the offside whilst the lead rope is in the hand of the wheelchair user. They need to learn to be followed by both the lines and the wheelchair if longlining from a wheelchair is to take place. To allow safe wheelchair working adequate staffing, clear understanding, well trained horses and ease of access to good floor surfaces are all needed. This is definitely an area in which a horse needs to have received specific training and shown themselves consistently suited to the work.

5.2.2 General fitness

Fitness is needed by a therapy horse engaged in ridden work of any kind but clearly not as much as in a competition horse. Indeed high levels of fitness can preclude work in therapy as the horse may be livelier and more reactive.

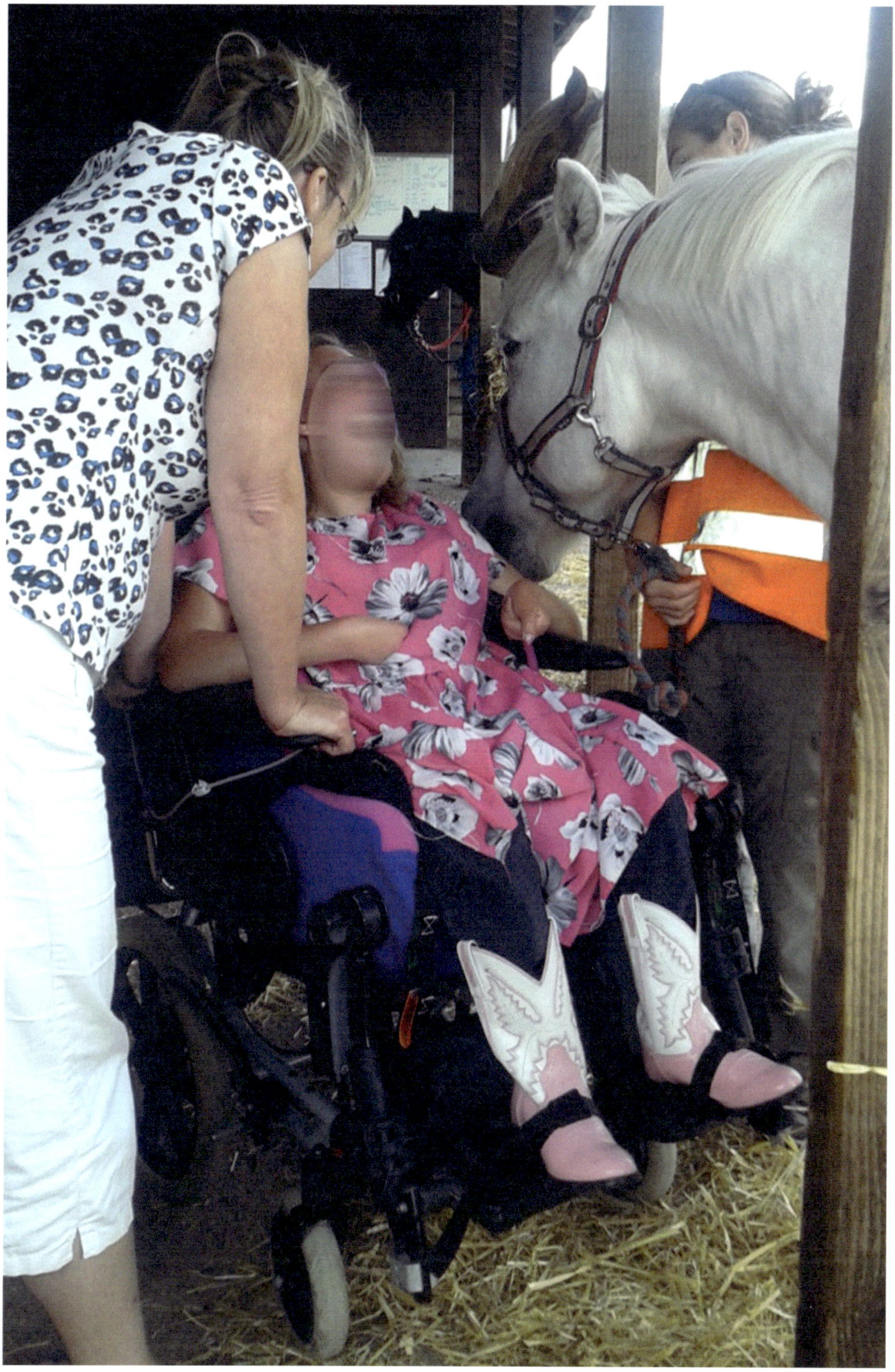

Image 16: Working with people using wheelchairs

Any new horse needs to be assessed on arrival and allowed to settle in. Then what it already knows can be established and also its ability to learn. The most important thing in this early period is to ensure it is handled by those who can correct any unhelpful behaviours so that issues don't arise later when it is being used in therapy. It would be sensible to appoint one experienced member of staff to get to know the horse before using it in therapeutic interventions. Horses will be more reactive when unsettled by change of herd, handler or role.

5.3 The care of the therapy horse

There are no short cuts to a good therapy horse and when one is found great care needs to be taken to maintain its health and well-being for the work.

Therapy horses should be trained in the roles for which they have been chosen. These may be several therapeutic roles or they may have a secondary role such as one in a mainstream riding school. Horses used in therapeutic interventions in which there is release of emotion need to have time to relax and this is best done through herd time. Stabling horses used in

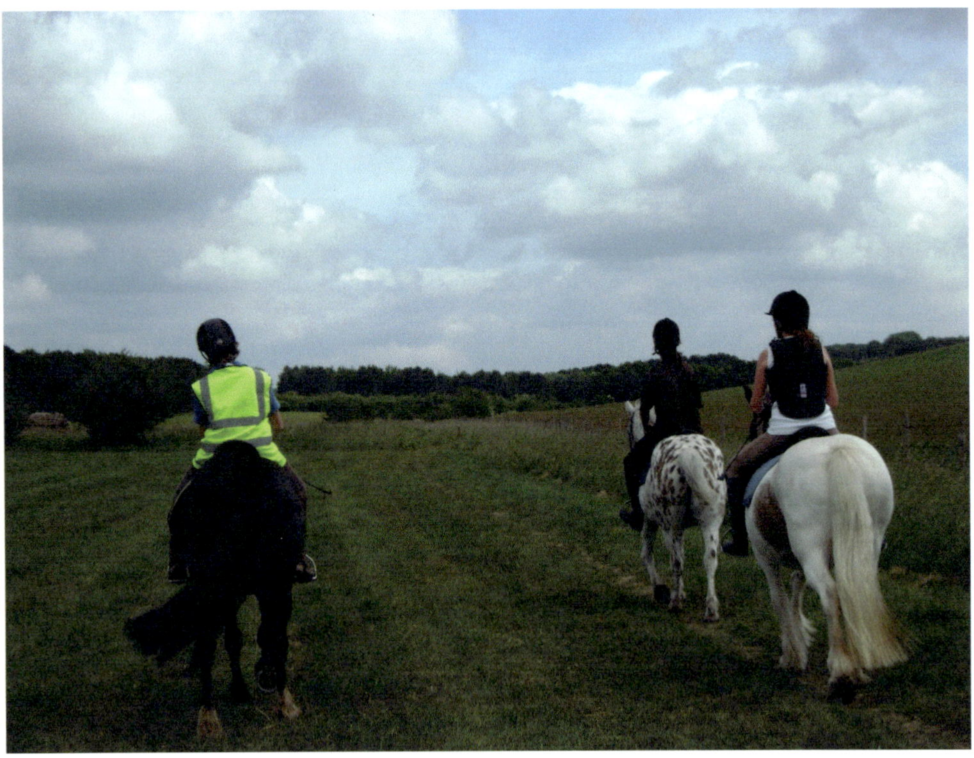

Image 17: Canter track ahead!

therapy is of course necessary at times, but animals which are free to roll, graze and groom with others stay fresher in the work than those who can not be part of the herd in this way.

Whatever their job is a horse benefits from learning something new or having an occasional week off. The opportunity for a change in role or a fast ride with a competent rider also help to prevent staleness.

The work done in carrying unlevel or unbalanced loads in physical therapy sessions can produce neck and back problems in the horse and care of this, alongside good saddle fitting, will help. All mounting can put pressure on the side of the horse even when a mounting block is used and if the rider is physically disabled this can be increased.

Horses used in such work need to ideally have two weight limits for their ridden work, one for well balanced riders and one for unbalanced ones.

The advantages of horses being barefoot in this work has already been mentioned and there is increasing research showing reduced incidence of lifetime lameness in the unshod, leading to more farriers now practising both farriery and equine podiatry.

Horses being used in therapy who have been rescued or retired to a therapy role need appropriate management of their condition. Extra care must be taken that the new role in therapy, which some incorrectly dismiss as being no effort for the horse, does not adversely affect them.

For a horse to be a good member of the team during therapy sessions it needs to be well known to the handler and generally contented. Such animals help provide safe and effective sessions so no effort made in the selection, training and care of these horses is ever wasted.

Case study 5

Melanie was a 14 year old girl brought to Gul by her mother. Her mother reported being distressed that she could not help her daughter adequately. Melanie had started doing very superficial self-harm, which was mostly cutting her forearms. Mother reported that Melanie seemed to find school work difficult and that Melanie's younger sister was slimmer, thought to be prettier by some, sporty and bright. Mother was trying a wide range of sensible possible actions and discovered that Melanie had some musical ability which Melanie was not prepared to invest in.

The girl's father had left some six years previously and mother had returned to work full time in a local school. Mother reported that the girls' weekend visits and holiday stays to their father were managed amicably. Mother was desperate to find her daughter some help and her friend had suggested Gul.

Melanie and her mother came to an assessment with a psychology trained volunteer. A good history was taken and advice on safer self-harming given to Melanie in line with harm reduction best practice. Then, whilst Melanie was being shown around the site by a member of staff, mother was given a little more advice on the approach to managing self-harm in a teenager.

The therapist ensured that Melanie was currently safe and knew what to do if she felt less safe, i.e. in danger of significant self-harm. She also made sure that Melanie did not have suicidal ideation. Melanie was clearly going through an adolescent phase of uncertainty, worried that she would have a poor relationship as she believed her parents had done, worried that she would not find a life partner and appeared to be ambivalent about being overweight and a little unattractive. She felt this made her safer from having relationships and yet, as is very common, really wanted to experience a relationship. The therapist had said little about this but suggested she got to know some of the ponies instead.

Melanie was invited back and was seen by a Level 1 trained member of staff, an Assistant Riding Coach with a naturally bubbly personality. This member of staff was chosen as she was a young female and a good role model for struggling teenagers. Her incessant jollity and chatter is able to cajole most into joining in. Melanie wasn't quite sure that she would like horses but quickly fell in love with MacDuff, the steady, ancient, 13.2 hand highland pony in the team. Her love for MacDuff was so evident, and her love of grooming and learning to ride so all-consuming, that it was not long before MacDuff was the photograph in the study book which she referred to when feeling stressed at school. Melanie found belonging and value through coming to Gul. Her physical activity levels went up and her need to comfort eat went down so her weight was also helped through these activities. With no special psychological input whatsoever, Melanie grew in confidence through learning to ride and she was enabled to succeed by taking and passing her ABRS weekly rider tests. She took part in the very small, in-house, Summer Show and gained several rosettes.

The improvement in Melanie's well-being simply from being involved in riding school activities had a wide impact. Her father, sister and school friends and teachers all registered the change.

When the time came for Melanie to leave school and move on to college, she lost touch with Gul but was safely re-established in mainstream education with an understanding of where she could go for help in the future.

Chapter 6

Measuring for success

6.0 The purpose of recording and measuring

To date there is very little information available on successful outcomes in this area of work from which to learn and from which further development can arise. Paradoxically this gives more value to the small amount of information that there is. The lack of a large volume of proof of successful outcomes is finally being addressed by research in this area.

Horses in Education and Therapy International (HETI) have a biannual peer reviewed journal which is a recent, and most welcome, addition to the libraries. University dissertations are available for reading as is much anecdotal writing but wider literature searches for peer reviewed work with large sample sizes still brings up comparatively few papers. This is not surprising if the area of Outdoor Therapy as a whole is only some fifty years old.

Return On Investment (ROI) is a widely used term in business and the return refers to the value that has been added by the process. The cost of producing that return is referred to as the investment. In an equine environment a suitable example might be that of building a new indoor school for the centre. Investment of time and money is needed to build the school and the increased revenue brought in by the increased activity made possible will be the return on the investment.

The investment of resources used in a therapy session will include money for general overheads, staff time and horse keep and the added value produced, the main return, is the improvement in the participant. There may also be increased income, including some profit, if the activity is fully funded.

Measurements and data which show improvement in participants are valuable to the therapists involved, the organisations in which they work, the person engaged in therapy, their family and carers, the referring agency (perhaps a school), the funder of the sessions and any banks or donors supporting the work financially.

Measurements and data are also very valuable to those who care for the horses as they can show how many hours a horse has worked and what type of work they have undertaken. The word "data" is used to mean the numerical records associated with the provision of therapy and this data both gives a value to the horse and informs management decisions.

The work and process involved in measuring should be kept as simple and effective as possible and integral to the sessions. If measuring is made into a main workstream of its own this can become a detrimental focus of activity.

In summary, data collection is undertaken to:-

- inform therapists and therapy teams, allowing continuous professional development
- prove to participants that progress is being made
- prove to funders that their money is making a difference
- show ROI to funders
- allow better management of resources
- show families and carers that the provision is making a difference
- record the horses' contribution
- show banks and donors that development plans are based on facts not dreams.

6.1 How to measure success

Measuring success is quite different to just measuring. Many things can be measured but if something is easy to measure it doesn't make it useful unless it is an important something. Measuring for success involves the identification and reliable collection of useful data preferably by a simple method, followed by data collation and analysis sufficient to give understanding.

In many walks of life there is a tendency to measure the easily measured rather than the important.

6.1.1 Useful data

Useful data is that which informs the therapist's next action, leads to improvement, demonstrates change in all areas and shows the contribution of the horse based therapy in a way that helps fund its future.

The changes demonstrated will be in the areas of physical, mental and emotional health, human behaviour, general wellbeing and education.

A new centre considering offering therapy needs to look at how it will record its activity and keep confidential any personal data gathered.

To measure change in anything there is a need to record the starting point so that the information gathered at the finishing point can be compared with it. Information gathered therefore needs to be:-

- reliable and reproducible
- accessible
- acceptable to those taking part and to their families and carers
- efficient in terms of the staff and participant time taken to gather and record it
- useable across the range of therapeutic interventions, regardless of complexity
- safely and easily stored with due regard to confidentiality
- externally validated as a method of information gathering if using a questionnaire

Examples of suitable questionnaires available online include:-

- The World Health Organisation Wellbeing Tool
- Assessment tools for mental health in adults such as psychological health questionnaire and generalised anxiety and depression scale
- General physiotherapy assessment tools and examples from other fields
- Analogue scale measurement.

Useful information is that which shows the investment and the return resulting from it, whether that return was improved core strength and walking after an accident, or improved mental health and returning to work after a crisis. The targets set are the goals of the therapy and are agreed before the start of sessions. The goals can of course be changed if the need changes as therapy develops, but to measure progress towards a goal is to measure for success. Goal setting is a well tried and tested method that will work in this area as in most areas of life whether aiming for a certain qualification or job or losing weight. The progress towards the goal, once measured, can enable the provision to be modified if needed.

6.1.2 The process of creating change -input to impact

In the previous section the resources needed to produce a therapy session were touched on and it is worth taking a moment to map a process with a view to data collection. The concept and understanding of a process can be used with examples across life from baking a cake to running a therapy session.

Input -the input to a process refers to that which is put into the process to make it happen. In the case of a horse based therapeutic intervention we know this to be money, time, the horse and the skill of the therapist. This has been referred to earlier as the investment. The input produces the output which is simply what the process delivers numerically. An input in a therapy centre would be, for example, 1 × 15 minute session using 2 staff and 1 horse for a school age person.

Output -the output is often likened to the production in a factory making widgets. If the product is widgets then measuring output is counting the widgets produced. The output in the example above would be one therapy session of 15 minutes.

Outcome -the outcome is wider than the output and includes all the subjectively felt effects caused by the process, even those felt by the referrer. This therefore includes characteristics beyond those measured in numbers alone. An improvement in how the person feels at the end of the session needs to be recorded and, if recorded in words alone, this can be used as anecdotal evidence of effect. If it is recorded as a numerical value by using a questionnaire at the start and end of a session or series of sessions the numerical difference can be used to more reliably demonstrate an effect.

Impact -The impact is the outcome taken wider still and is harder to demonstrate. One of the reasons for this is that the impact of the process can take time to develop. Measuring impact in therapy requires a prospective, or forward looking, approach to data collection such as revisiting the recipient's life six months after starting therapy or perhaps six months after completing therapy. The experiences of the person prior to therapy, such as ten days lost from work to illness per month, would have been recorded as the reason for attending the centre. If this figure has reduced to five days per month then the impact of the therapy has been felt by the employer and the local economy as well as the recipient and funder.

If a therapeutic intervention influences someone's behaviour, their self confidence and life plan, this may lead to less police time used in managing their misdemeanours over the following years so benefitting society as a whole. The person may be able to be employed rather than being on benefits and give a more stable home to their young family thereby improving outcomes for the future generation too. This impact is therefore felt by society as a whole, but measuring this will necessarily take many years.

The measurement and data collection undertaken by any centre should be targeted to show the input, or investment of resources, and the progress in the areas of output, outcome and impact as the return on the investment.

As horse based therapy is more expensive than some alternative therapies the provider needs to demonstrate increased effectiveness over other less expensive interventions in order to justify the increased cost of its use.

6.1.3 Quantitative and qualitative data

The two main categories of data used to show output and outcome are quantitative and qualitative, which are also known as hard and soft data respectively.

Quantitative data is hard data and numerical whilst qualitative is soft data, not numbers based but rather characteristic based, and therefore is harder to measure. Examples of qualitative data would be improved self-confidence or increased resilience in the person engaged in therapy.

Quantitative measurements are not difficult to create or manage. It is simply recording what took place in terms of the input and output and is purely numbers based. Quantitative measurements at a therapeutic centre should show the hours of therapy given using headings from the matrix, the numbers of people helped and the hours taken in the process. The age group of the people and the high level classification of the disadvantages seen is helpful to give the picture of the activity undertaken. The numbers gathered should show input and output and be recorded, collated, analysed and stored safely.

Qualitative measurements include questionnaires, diaries, anecdotal stories (with no personal identifiable details), interviews, focus groups and observations. To make these measurements the therapist, therapy assistant or therapy team need good interpersonal skills and to have planned and prepared prior to the session. The need is to be clear about what is to be measured and what the goals of the therapy are. It is important to have the relevant paperwork to hand in advance.

Qualitative measurements, the soft outcomes, can be straightforward ones such as measuring mood improvement using a nationally accredited tool such as Generalised Anxiety and Depression Scale (GADS) at the start and end of the session. When the soft outcome is not straightforward to measure a proxy indicator may be needed.

6.1.4 Proxy indicators

If an agreed soft outcome or goal seems too abstract to measure a set of proxy indicators will be useful. These are indicators that can demonstrate the soft outcome chosen even if it is something that can't be directly measured. Indicators are subjective when the person engaged in therapy gives their opinion of change or, alternatively, the indicators are objective when the opinion is given by someone else. This may be the opinion of the therapist, therapy assistant or external person such as the school teacher or carer of the person.

Proxy indicators vary depending on what is to be evaluated and are usually themselves measured in an analogue scale with a linear, numerical approach. An analogue scale is a way of measuring subjective characteristics or attitudes, ranging across a continuum that cannot be directly measured.

EXAMPLE
A teenager with low self-confidence comes to the yard for therapy. Let us call the teenager Frank.

During the assessment you are tempted to give up and not offer sessions because Frank will hardly speak to you. His mother reports he is monosyllabic at home as well. Frank's views about anything are hard to elicit as his normal monosyllabic phase as a teenager is compounded by shyness and the fear that follows him. The young person looks at the ground whilst walking or talking, he gives no voluntary eye contact and hides behind his overlong fringe.

Frank looks as if he is trying to be invisible. He is. He would rather be anywhere else. He looks awkward throughout, hands in pockets. His clothing is unremarkable and dark in colour. Sessions are agreed and begin but he is rarely on time for them. Mother explains that this is because she can't easily get him to come.

As a Level 1 centre you are not concerning yourself with the background to the loss of confidence, simply to restoring it to a natural level for his age. All manner of horse care offered at the centre will be useful but as already discussed belonging, value and success based interventions are the best ones to use for Frank.

Proxy indicators for Frank's self-confidence would be set. The indicators would be chosen to measure improvement in the young person's behaviour towards the accepted norm for their age. In this case the expected norm would probably be to stand tall, walk with their head up, talk to people met without mumbling, be on time most of the time, give good eye contact and make less use of the fringe. Each indicator would be given an analogue scale and a standard recovery star is an excellent tool for measuring this, see Fig. 18.

Another example of the use of proxy indicators is to measure change in emotion or feeling such as anger, low mood, fear or anxiety. Therapy teams will learn to be creative with proxy indicators as they become familiar with using them if not already doing so. Proxy indicators that may be useful are:-

- initiating conversation
- replying in more than one word or phrase
- changing clothes colour
- trying something new
- walking into a room first
- going somewhere alone
- using public transport

- argument reduction in a relationship
- activities carried out successfully with other people

Clearly the list is neither long nor exhaustive but intended to show the possibilities given by proxy indicators in measuring soft outcomes of therapy.

6.1.5 Recovery star

A standard recovery star allows overall goals or proxy indicators to be measured at the start of a course of therapy sessions and remeasured at a set number of weeks to evaluate the improvement.

Fig. 18: Blank Recovery Star

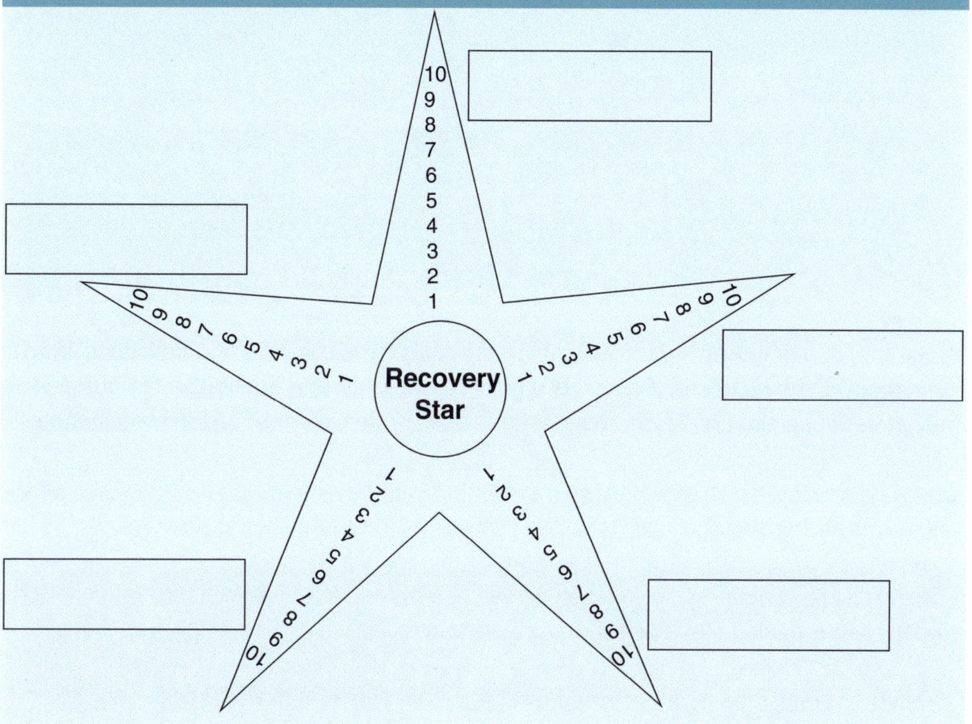

A recovery star could list goals such as:-

- riding as a sport, aiming to achieve Level 4 Association of British Riding School test
- improved self confidence
- improved attendance at school
- reduction in health care attendances
- walking with no aid

Fig. 19: Recovery Star for Frank

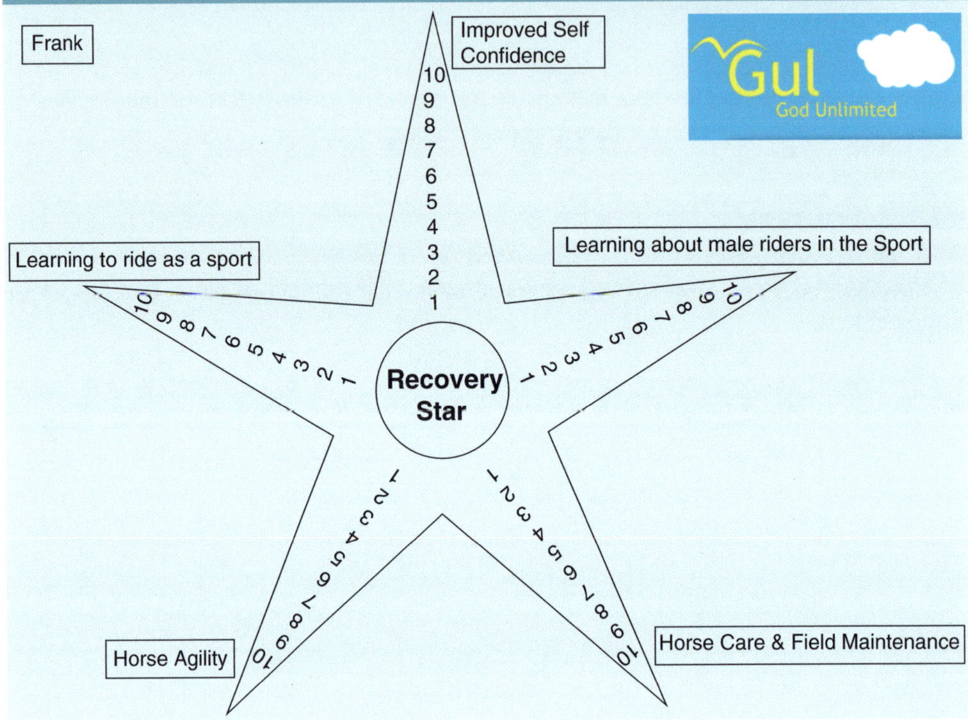

At the start of therapy, after the assessment, the goals are set and are of course done with the agreement of the recipient. If a goal is difficult to measure and qualitative in nature, proxy indicators are agreed and in the above list this clearly refers to improved self confidence.

One way of recording this qualitative information is to have a second recovery star for this area alone and writing the aspects to be measured at the spokes of the star.

The starting level on all spokes is then agreed as a numerical value with the recipient of the therapy and reviewed after the set amount of input to see what, if anything, has changed.

To return to Frank for a moment we could agree a star with him that looked like Fig. 19.

Due to the need to show improvement in self confidence via proxy indicators we could also agree a star for that which might look like Fig. 20.

After an agreed amount of time the stars are reviewed and the analogue scales revisited and the two circles can then be compared and the data recorded as shown below.

The use of recovery stars is easy, is already widespread and the findings nationally understood. The initial completion of, or revisiting of, stars does not need to take much time but is 10 minutes well invested in the future of both the person and the centre.

Fig. 20: Proxy Indicator Recovery Star for self confidence

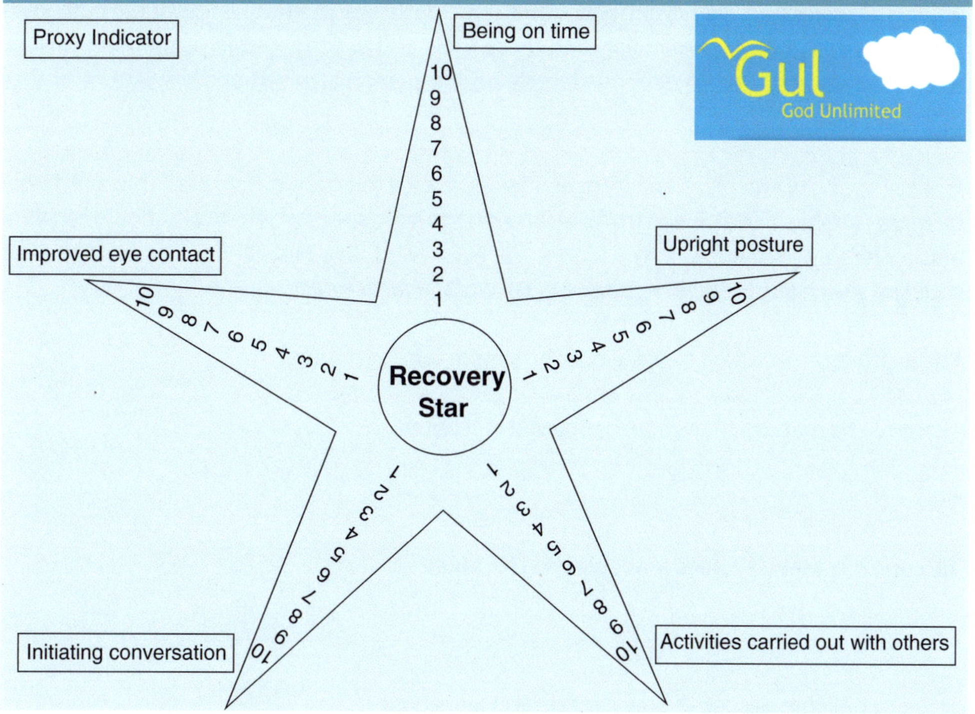

Fig. 21: Frank's Proxy Indicator Star at the end of the course

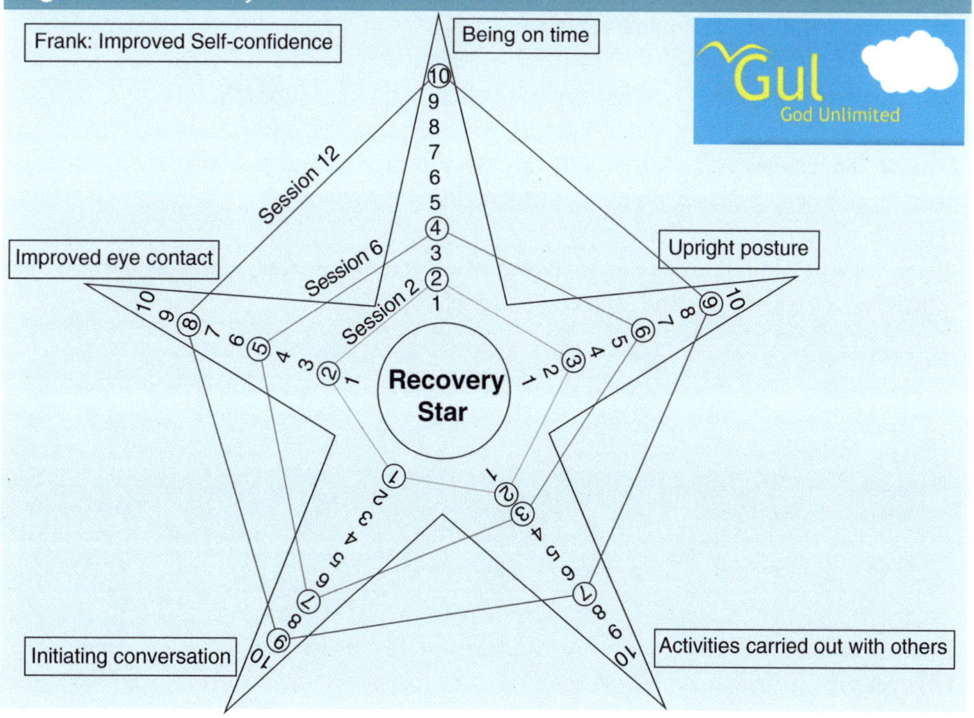

6.1.6 Analogue scales

Analogue scales can be verbal and visual and both are useful in measuring outcomes. Therapists will already be familiar with these tools and experienced in using them to good effect. The choice of scale depends largely on the person involved and the nature of their disadvantage.

Whilst a recovery star gives one form of analogue scale there are others available which may be more suitable. If the person involved is on the autistic spectrum the scale should be visual and preferably with boxes into which a tick is inserted. See Fig. 22. Each end of the scale could be given simply and in writing, e.g. 0 = worst and 10 = best.

The instruction on where to tick would be simple too, for example:-

Tick one box that describes how happy you feel about …

or

Tick one box that describes how safe you feel about …

or

Tick one box that describes how content you feel about …

If the person taking part has a learning difficulty or has trouble concentrating a visual scale with pictures and colours could be useful (Fig. 23).

Now the person in therapy is asked to circle or tick with verbal support.

If the person is better verbally than with any other form of communication they can be asked to estimate where they now placed themselves using the sentence:

"If you were at 2 in terms of self-confidence when you first started, where would you place yourself now if 0 was none and 10 is very self confident?"

Fig. 22: Analogue Scale 1

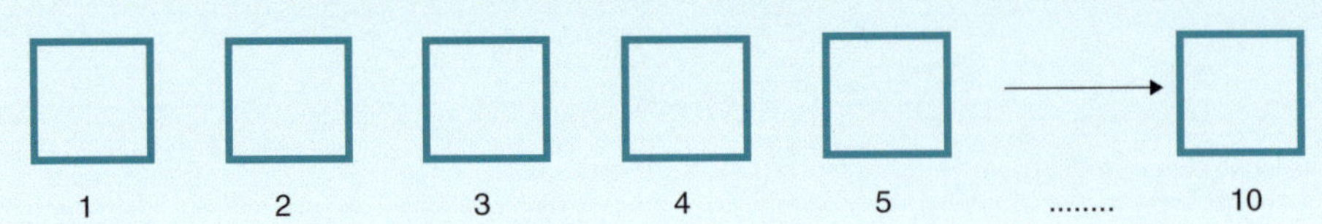

Fig. 23: Analogue Scale 2

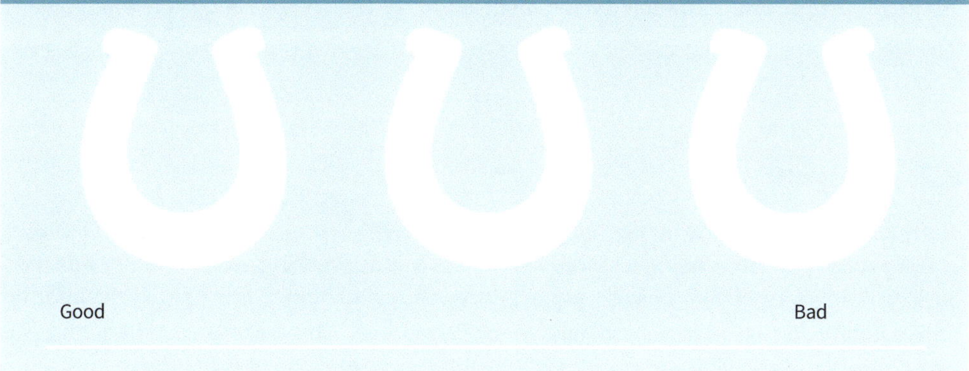

6.1.7 Triangulation

For anyone in a therapeutic setting who is having difficulty with the tools a family member or carer could assist. To do this they would need to be adequately aware of the process underway. The use of family and carers can be put to good effect in the process of triangulation.

Triangulation is taken from a navigation technique when 3 viewpoints are used to confirm a geographical position.

When used in a therapy setting to confirm a person's position on a scale three opinions are used and an average value attributed. The three opinions may not overlap precisely but give a confident overall assessment. The opinions would commonly be the person involved in the therapy, a family member or carer, and the therapist or therapy assistant. This method often has the advantage of sparking discussion which is beneficial to all involved.

6.1.8 Journeying

For some people, their progress is best described in terms of journeying. This will apply usually to adults with some life behind them. It is helpful for those who have had support of various types in the past but slipped back into old ways. Expecting a nice, clean and tidy 6 week solution for them is neither realistic nor helpful.

In a River of Life, freely available on the internet, the person notes or draws events or milestones in their life. These may be positive and enabling events with good memories or negative ones, i.e. obstacles. These milestones have happened along their journey on the river of life and have made them who they are today or brought them to this place. The recipient then, with the help of the therapist, prepares steps or stages for the journey ahead. They may identify things that have been in their way in the past that they need to work on and decide what the end of the next stage of the journey looks like. In this way progress along the river can be judged.

Passing stages on the journey, or moving up the analogue scale on the recovery star, allows the therapist, the team and the person involved to be encouraged and motivated towards success.

6.2 Analysis

Analysis of collected data is essential. It takes time and can be seen as an administrative activity easily put off as being less important. It is a good working practice to provide feedback on hard and soft outcomes on a quarterly basis as a minimum and to have the information regularly discussed at Senior Manager or Board level. This will ensure it happens, is fit for its purpose of showing success and will thereby underpin a successful future.

In financially constrained times which seem likely to prevail for some years, it will be hard to produce good, well informed, business cases for funding in horse based therapy. The outcomes of the therapeutic interventions must be well documented and there is no shortcut available for this. Measuring for success requires application but it is well worth making this effort.

6.3 Why measure?

When the issue of measuring is discussed it is often talked about in a negative way and as an unwelcome action imposed by others. It is as if data collection holds no value. Initially there may be little interest shown in data by those involved in providing therapeutic interventions.

This is incorrect. The understanding that data brings is invaluable and therefore should be of great interest to all involved. The time and effort taken to measure, collate and understand the data gathered ensures resources are used wisely. It also has the potential to demonstrate progress towards goals whether to therapists, recipients or funders. A lack of data and the understanding that it brings means that decisions may appear to be based on little more than guesswork.

Much of the information available in this field is based on anecdotal evidence and few large scale studies have been undertaken. If horse based therapy becomes more widely available the potential for collecting larger volumes of data on larger numbers of recipients becomes possible. This will, of course, be easier if similar data collection systems are used in all centres, perhaps by using that which is outlined above. Larger studies would then form the basis of useful research into the effectiveness of this work.

This chapter has concentrated on measuring for success in terms most relevant to an Outdoor Therapy Centre and its provision but record keeping and measuring in general is essential for research, both now and in the future.

Case study 6

Richard is 5 years old and has Down's Syndrome. He comes to Gul with his brother who does not have any recognised disadvantage. They take part together in a shared family activity and both boys benefit. Richard's disadvantage is not particularly severe although at times he cannot listen to instructions if he is very excited. This led, one day, to Richard walking with the girth right under the horses belly to do it up on the other side. Thankfully, the well chosen and very calm pony stood completely still showing no response to this experience. It only happened once!

Mother reported that after riding sessions at Gul, Richard was calmer and more able to relax. This was put down to the mindfulness approach produced by a quiet half hour hack on a pony whose movement called him back to the present. Mother reported that, in her opinion, the improvement caused by the riding lasted three days into the following week.

The family continued to attend for several years until moving away from the area. They were subsequently in touch with the charity reporting their delight at being able to go riding as a family at a Trekking Centre when on holiday in Cornwall.

Horses had helped Richard's physical health, his emotional wellbeing and had impacted the whole family by removing the apparent barrier of disadvantage. They had been able to be a family group on holiday.

Chapter 7

Moving on to practise safely

In this final chapter the information is drawn together so that it can be used for its intended purpose: to enable a competent, professional, horse based therapy programme to be developed and provided.

If the preceding chapters have provoked interest in the provision of horse assisted therapy, or in changing the provision already in place, one aim of the book has been met. In order to keep the practice safe, however, there are further factors to consider. These are explored in this chapter before the pathway is explained.

To practise safely there is a need to look beyond the session itself to the supporting structures which underpin provision.

7.0. The team

Team is a much used word but working as a team is an acquired skill and not a natural process. Teams are usually made up of people but in the case of horse based therapy the horse could also be considered a member. A team is defined as:-

“A group of people with different skills and shared values working towards a common goal.”

A good team has members whose individual skills complement each other. In other words a good team is not necessarily made from people who are similar and are friends with each other. A good team will have a selection of different skills and personalities within it so the ability of the team to achieve its goals is widened. With diversity comes the challenge of working together well.

Teamworking has been tried and tested in many different settings over the years and there is a profusion of literature and teaching material available on the subject. Teamworking is widely used because it is effective. When a team is working well it enhances the productivity of the group due in part to the commitment within the team providing a synergistic effect. Teamworking is also known to promote resilience in team members and so adds to the resilience of the service provision.

7.0.1 An effective team

An effective team works hard at working together because being an effective team is not easy, but common principles of working in this way are:-

- to value all the members
- to know the skills of all of the team members and how they are best used
- to have a shared vision and goals
- to know who the team leader is at any one time
- to have a set of agreed team rules
- to know how to resolve conflict
- to communicate well

Team rules can be helpful and might include being on time for meetings or sessions, not leaving until everyone has finished work, listening before speaking and supporting each other. Ideally the rules are decided by the team and setting the rules can in itself be a formative experience for the new team.

Communication was discussed in the expansion of the matrix. It is important to use the most efficient ways of communicating so that, for example, precious time is not wasted by driving to meetings when a phone call or video call would suffice.

7.0.2 Building a team

Building a team takes time and the first step is to ensure that there is a shared vision, understood by all and a recognition that the team is valuable to the organisation as a whole.

The leadership of a team needs to be clear but can certainly change as the team undertakes different stages of tasks to deliver the goal. The team leader could be decided by the team but is most often chosen by the overall manager of the organisation.

Growing ownership of any process is helped by enabling the team members to set the goals they are aiming for. The provision of an Offer Matrix and recovery stars for individual recipients will aid this process. The growing team needs to learn things together, decide up on and keep to its rules and ensure that time is made available for meeting as a team.

Teams need to be built according to the role they will have and the part they will play in the outcomes of the organisation. This may seem obvious but teams that struggle are those with square pegs in round holes and this happens when the "you'll do" is applied at times of low staff resource.

Teams can also struggle if there is too high a proportion of one skill or personality type leaving those that don't easily match it feeling uncomfortable or left out.

Whilst provision always remains a priority, a less developed team or an unbalanced team will not be as effective. An example would be a team made up of the remnants of several other teams during the summer leave season.

A useful exercise for building a team is to practise new skills on colleagues or other team members, that will be needed prior to working with actual recipients of therapy.

7.0.3 The centre's team

Here the "team" refers to those who work together in a centre. It may, therefore, mean that the people working at a riding centre consider adding therapeutic interventions at Level 1. This team would include riding coaches, office staff, grooms, helpers, and handyman alike. In a team no one is "just" an anything. Whether answering the phone with a smile, ensuring all paperwork is ready, or preparing the horse for its role, the tasks need to be done well and all contribute to the outcome of the session.

A therapist or therapy assistant discovering that the horse isn't tacked up correctly will be frustrated or stressed by the delay and feel let down by the team, leading to a less effective intervention for those attending. Similarly, a grumpy groom can unsettle a horse before it starts to work and this will detract from the potential effectiveness of the intervention. Knowing the personality and behaviours of those in the team simply improves the overall outcome by using everyone's own areas of strength.

For example, the bouncy, friendly and chatty riding coach may not work best for people with autistic spectrum disorder but may be ideal for the anxious or ADHD rider. Similarly, if a team member has had negative experiences with alcoholic parents and/or neglect in childhood which is as yet unprocessed they are unlikely to be able to help with a session involving these issues. They may even be affected enough by the triggering of personal memories to require help themselves. This does not mean that they could not help effectively in other therapy settings.

In Chapter 3 the choice and care of horses was considered as was the importance of knowing them well. Any horse can behave "out of character" at times but knowing what they usually bring to a session is essential. It allows the therapist or therapy assistant to choose the horse most likely to help produce the desired change. This is routine work for anyone involved with horses. Placing the rider on the correct horse for a lesson is a commonly practised skill at riding centres and every experienced horse owner knows exactly how to keep their horse and rider safe whilst offering a ride to a friend or relative. Leading reins have been used over the centuries for just such a reason.

Once the horse team member is chosen for a session the therapist or therapy assistant needs sufficient understanding to use the horse / human interaction to increase the effectiveness of the therapeutic intervention. Without this they may as well be practising generic outdoor therapy and using a bicycle or a map and compass.

Occasionally, in purely physical therapy, a therapist or therapy assistant may know enough about the movement of the horse in general to guide the session. Whilst they manage the therapy the horse leader's task is to be aware of the horse's comfort, alertedness and any other equine issues. The therapist is thereby free to concentrate on the recipient and the therapy. However if the therapist doesn't see that a horse is stiffer on one rein they will not realise the effect this will have on the rider's body, nor that the effect will be less than expected when using a bareback exercise. The overall outcome of the session will be affected.

The choice of the horse for such a session needs to be made in discussion with the horse skilled person on the team.

7.1 The self

Educators on teamwork love to quote that "There is no I in team" however they often miss the fact that there still is "me". Teams are built of individuals. The understanding of "self" for each team member allows the team to be built properly as each member has a "self " which will exert an effect within the team as a whole.

The understanding of self is useful for everyone and not just for team members about to provide therapeutic interventions. There is a great deal written about the subject and freely available on line. Before the team is built it is important for all team members to understand the concept of self.

Understanding oneself before engaging in any sort of therapeutic intervention is not difficult and should be undertaken to prevent surprises along the way. Work on personal self-awareness is part of preparation for work in any psychology field.

The reason is threefold.

Firstly, in order to enable change in people an understanding of how people behave is needed and a good way of achieving this is to use oneself as a working example. Secondly, the personal response felt to wards others can be better understood. Thirdly, understanding oneself will protect against subject matter disclosed during a session provoking difficult memories in a therapist or an assistant during a session.

Aspects of social psychology would suggest that knowledge of self can be assisted by understanding of the following:-

- personality type
- thinking style
- age
- life experience
- good balance in the 7 areas of life / personal resilience
- perception of self

If someone has never looked at this for themselves they may be surprised at what they learn when they do.

7.1.1 Personality type

There are several models of personality typing available on the internet and, whilst these are fairly simplistic, they would be sufficient to give an overview of the people working together in that team. Most readers will be aware of the terms extrovert or introvert. They may not be aware that in self-awareness terms this is to do with where people are energised from and not so much about whether they like parties or not.

There are always people we meet in everyday life with whom it feels easy to communicate and strike up a relationship and there are others who do not attract. This is probably due to personality type and will be no different when considering routine attendees at centres. If, however, a person with no disadvantage attending a riding centre for a lesson annoys the coach intensely it would be helpful to understand why. By understanding the response produced, the coach will be able to regain self-control and return to being professional without being stressed by the annoying (as perceived by them) behaviour. Sometimes a move to a different coach's session is all that is needed as what is annoying to one personality type will not necessarily be so to another.

7.1.2 Age

Younger people, and teenagers in particular, tend to be very polarised in their thinking and behaviour. They tend to see the world in black and white terms whereas older people can accept that shades of grey are common and actually useful. Once passed middle years the drive to personally succeed is usually accomplished and people become more tolerant and are more easily able to compromise. Clearly these are sweeping statements and can only be understood reviewing Fig. 4 describing the curve of normal distribution for anything. The overview of studying of the self given here is to encourage those who have not yet undertaken this to explore it further as it will assist their understanding of others as well as an understanding of themselves.

7.1.3 Life experience

Previous experiences in life affect expectations of outcome. If every time a child looks for praise they are belittled they learn to expect this. If every time someone loses a significant amount of weight they then put it back on, they come to expect this pattern to continue. If the last bus trip that they made involved a crash they may expect this to happen again. If the last horse they rode bolted and caused them to fall off, they may need time to regain their confidence and understanding that accidents can happen but do not always happen. The longer an experience has been reinforced, or the resulting behaviour has been in place, the longer it is going to take to change and the newly formed team needs to be aware of this.

They also need to be aware of how their own life experiences, both positive and negative, affect their behaviour today and how life experiences disclosed by others may trigger personal memories. These should not be ignored and must be dealt with, but this should be after the intervention has finished. The session is for the recipient, not for the team member.

7.1.4 Good life balance

Understanding that which gives balance in life is a useful tool. It is used in psychological therapies and it needs to be seen in team members lives too. There are various models available for this ranging from the complex to the simple. Balance is about well-being and considers time spent in exercise, in growing relationships, in personal skill growth as well as time spent on hobbies to ensure the individual remains healthy.

The classic example of lack of balance is that of addictive activity behaviour such as online gambling or gaming when individuals spend increasing amounts of time on the pursuit to the exclusion of sleep, exercise, talking to others and their ability to perform at work. This is an extreme example but serves to explain the concept.

7.1.5 Perception of self

How people see themselves is fascinating. Those with low self-esteem may see themselves as a liability in any activity and those who are over confident may actually be a liability. Here horse based work shows one of its strongest effects, that of enabling perception of self to be re-evaluated through the eyes of the horse, or rather by understanding the horse's emotional response to the human.

Understanding the self is clearly a large subject. Those without previous knowledge would benefit from observing a session or two at a Level 2 or 3 psychology based centre. Whether for oneself or for the team, time spent doing this would be an excellent investment.

7.2 Matrix and boundaries

This short section starts the process of mapping a centre's offer as provider. This is useful for the centre itself, for the team, for funders and for purchasers.

The first step is to decide on the level of the offer that the centre can make.

All riding centres could be Level 1 providers of therapeutic interventions. Under these circumstances the centre would work to a plan devised and supervised by an off site professional, who may be the referrer of the recipient.

A Level 2 centre will have a qualified physical health or psychology professional and would be able to deal with physical, mental and behavioural or emotional issues in their field of expertise as well as Level 1 interventions in other fields.

A centre with a professional team crossing the boundaries of physical, mental and behavioural disadvantages would be a Level 3 centre and able to manage complex cases.

The second step is to decide on the therapeutic interventions that can be offered at the centre.

The therapeutic interventions offered will be directly dependent upon the level of the centre and whether a Level 2 centre is based on physical or psychological therapy. Level 1 riding centres would be able to offer therapeutic interventions 1-5 on the matrix. Level 2 centres would be able to offer 1-5 plus 6 and either 7 or 8.

Level 3 centres would be able to offer all areas.

The third step is to decide on the areas of activity that the centre can offer.

The consideration of the areas of activity offered in the centre's matrix would include the site and the horses available for the work. A centre with one Shetland pony and some fields can certainly offer a great deal but clearly Riding as a Sport would only be possible for the short and light weight rider and only then if an appropriately qualified coach and safe space was available.

When a centre's team has confirmed that their collective awareness and insight is adequately developed, the team will be well placed to confirm its offer in terms of Horse Based Therapy. This can then be easily shown by creating the centre's offer matrix. It is suggested that a centre's offer matrix holds the full matrix but the areas unavailable are indicated as such, perhaps by grey background shading. The reason for this is that potential funders can make an informed choice to stay with the centre or be signposted to another with greater provision. It shows the position of the centre's level clearly so ensuring no one could claim they had been confused at the time of agreement. It is a good method of keeping a centre safe from criticism of its provision.

The use of the matrix makes the offer clear so the team member who wants to help everyone, and many teams will have one such member, may be aware of the centre's boundaries or limitations.

Boundaries are essential for maintaining the sustainability of the provision. A team that over extends itself and practises at the very edge of its competency may not stay in provision as the effectivity of what is offered will be reduced and some risks will be increased.

The simple analogy is that of a riding centre trying to teach competition showjumping in a muddy, slippery paddock. This will not work. The best approach is to set the level of delivery to that in which the centre's competency and strength will be demonstrated. Effective therapy outcomes will be the best way to impress. Over extension also threatens the resilience of the team itself so provision within the offer matrix should be set at a sustainable level.

It is often the case that a centre providing therapy does so at certain times only and this needs to be considered in order to keep all who come safe. Bringing someone with anxiety for a session at the same time as after school children's rides may precipitate behaviour that takes staff away from the children's activity to assist. If there is limited staff resource at certain times because other work is taking precedence, it is sensible to offer less provision. The temptation to push on despite difficulties should be avoided as this is when mistakes happen.

A centre should feel free to decline any request, simply giving a reason for so doing. The centre should be ready to signpost to other provision at this point using a previously gained understanding of what is provided locally. This allows the refusal to seem positive and makes for a helpful outcome to the enquirer.

Sustainability for self, family, team and horses is essential for today's therapy providers as the ever increasing demands and expectations of people can wear down reserves and cause mental, physical and system fatigue. A team should be good at looking for signs of overload within its members.

7.3 The emergency dismount

For centres working with epileptic patients, or patients suffering drop attacks of any kind or patients with hysterical behaviour, the therapy team needs to be trained in the art of safely dismounting the unconscious, possibly fitting, patient. This must be done without damage to rider, horse or staff. There is always the risk of a mounted fit, faint or episode being precipitated whilst on the horse, due to being paid more attention, being more relaxed or being more excited than usual. A centre working with such ridden sessions needs to carefully consider staffing ratios.

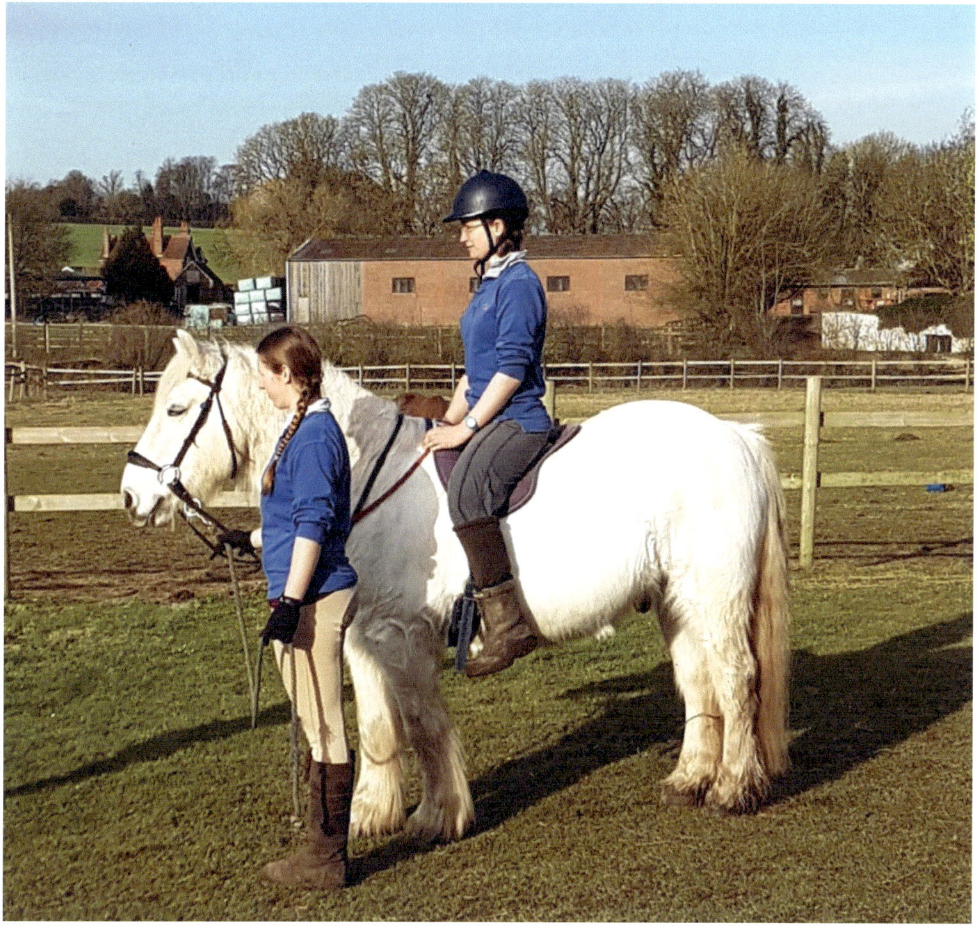

Emergency dismount 1: All is well

Such riders need to have one person assigned to them at all times and a second person within easy call distance e.g. in the same arena or field. This is likely to mean there is a leader and a therapist for all such sessions. It may be that the recipient has other disadvantages which would mean staffing support needs to be further increased, therefore having a leader and a side walker as well as the therapist.

The phases of the emergency dismount are as given below:-

1. The leader or therapist notices there is a problem.
2. The leader stops the horse, moves to its shoulder and assists the rider to lie forwards

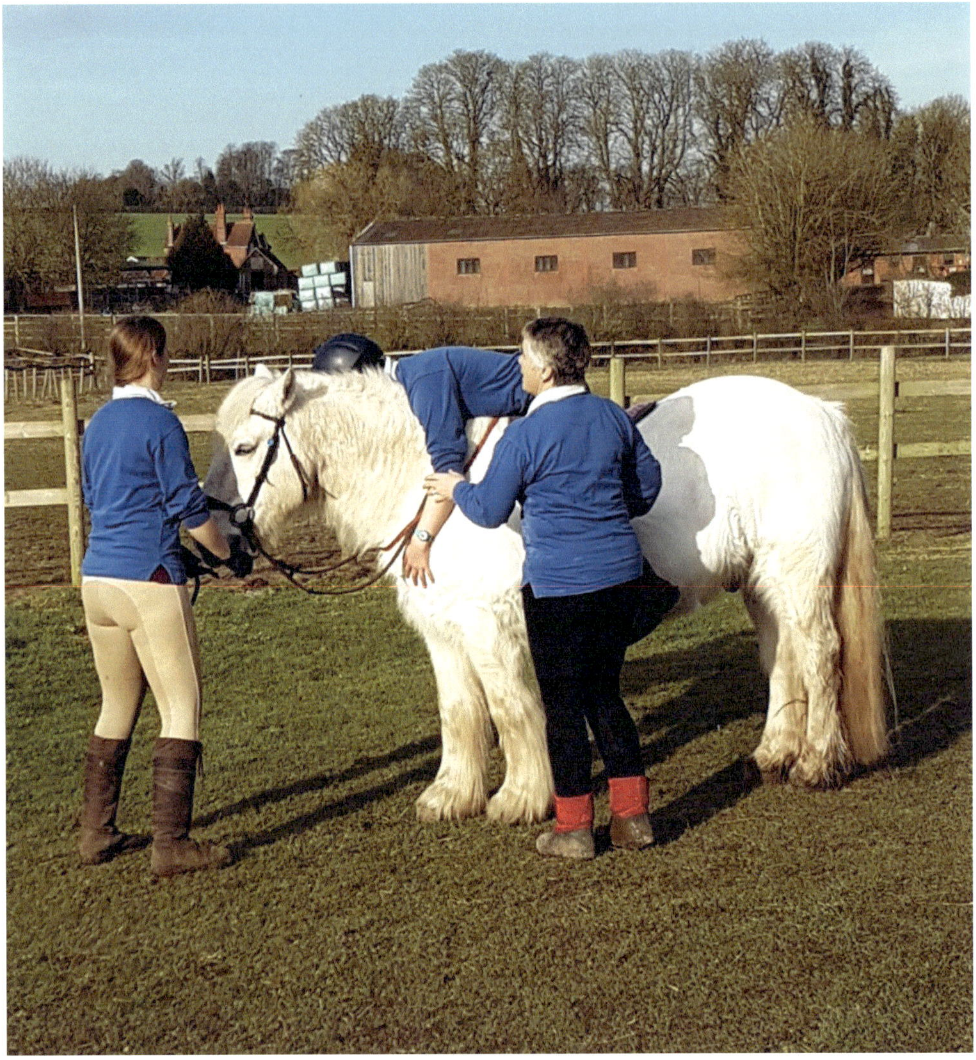

Emergency dismount 2: The second person arrives and the rider lies along the neck

on the horse's neck. The leader shouts for help.

3. The second person arriving goes to the left leg of the rider and the leader moves to the head of the horse to reassure and control it.
4. The second person at the riders leg reassures the rider, "Lie down, lie down and we will help you. You are quite safe." The second person at the rider's left leg keeps the rider lying forwards onto the horse's neck until a third person arrives.
5. The third person, depending on experience, either takes over the left leg of the rider

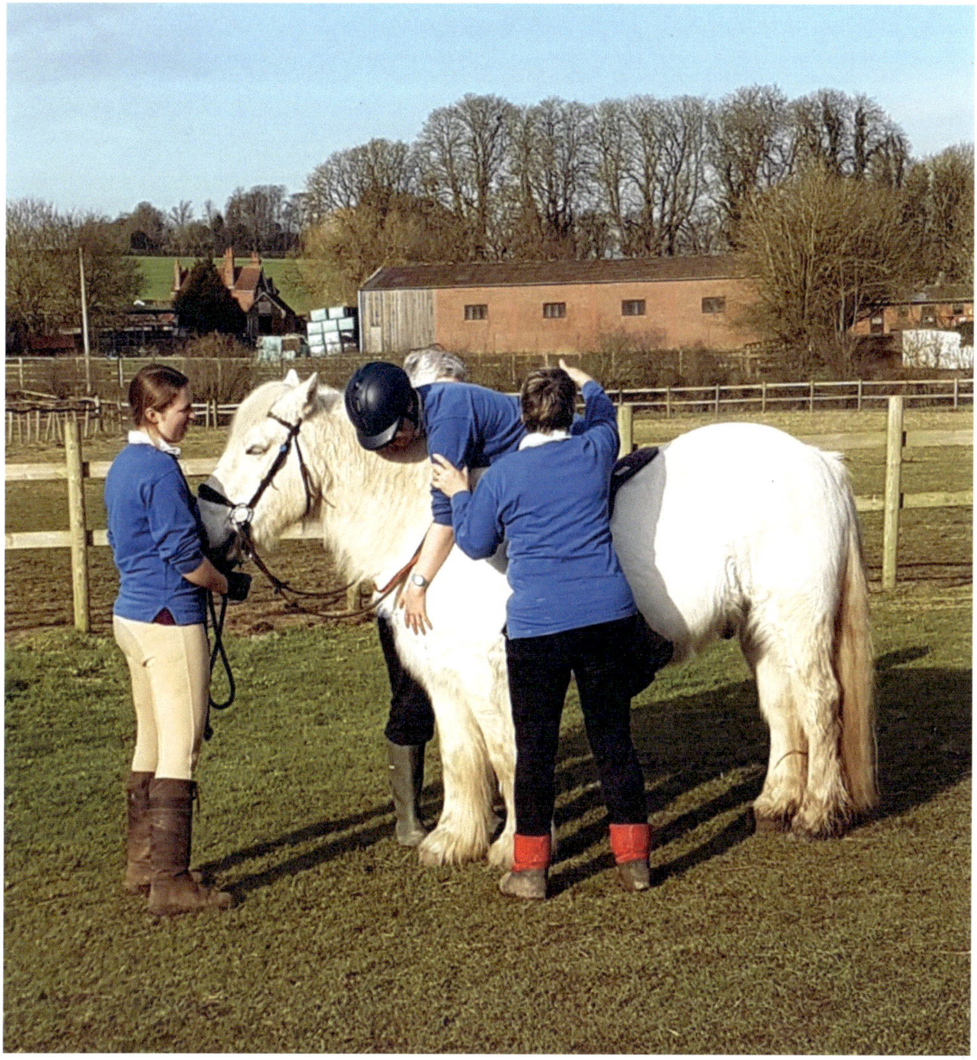

Emergency dismount 3: All are ready so the rider's feet come out of the stirrups

to control the descent or moves to the right leg of the rider. During this time the rider is reassured whether apparently conscious or not.

6. When all three people are in place, the left side one says "feet out" and both feet are removed from the stirrups. This can be difficult if tonic clonic seizures are taking place. If it is impossible to manage this the people on each side need to try to undo the stirrup leather buckle so the stirrup leather and iron can pull through and come off with the foot on dismounting. I have never known this to be needed but offer it in case of unusual circumstance.
7. The near side person decides whether there is enough room for the dismount

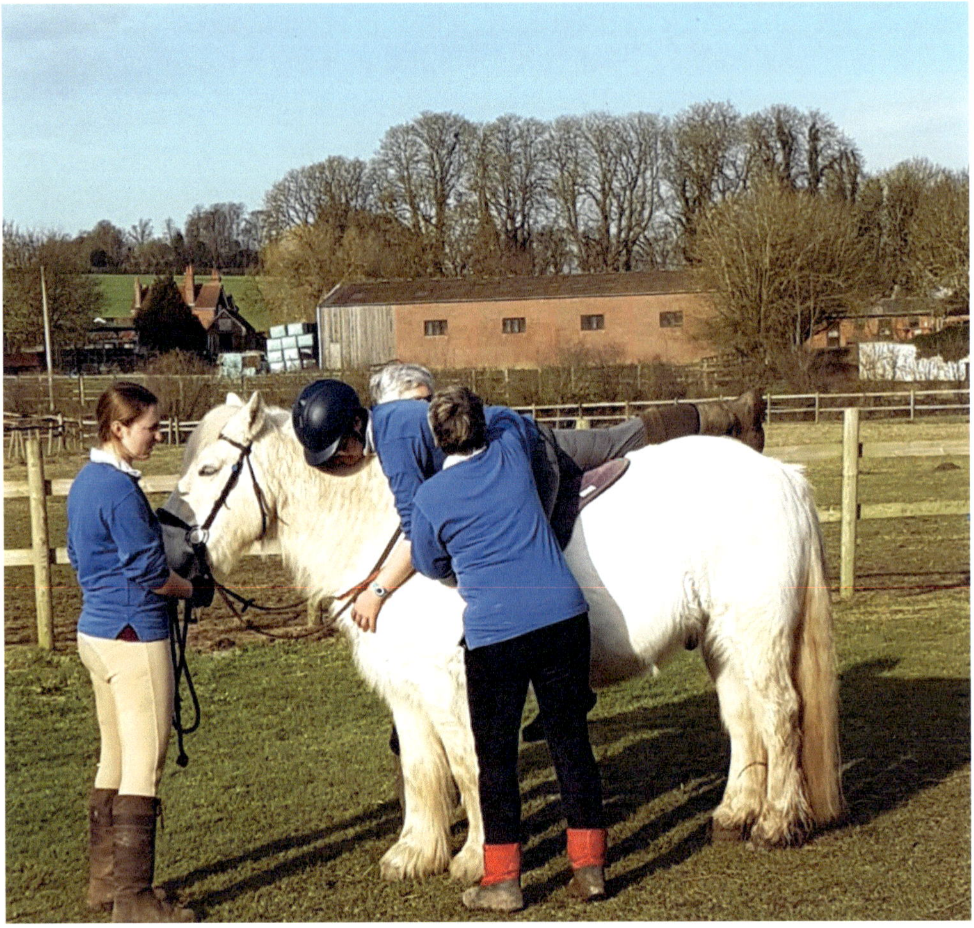

Emergency dismount 4: The right leg is lifted up from the offside

manoeuvre and advises moving the horse if not.

8. With the rider still lying along the neck of the horse the right leg is lifted backwards and upward imitating the movement of the dismounting swing of the right leg.
9. The near side person wraps their arms around the torso of the rider as soon as they are able. This depends on the size of the horse.
10. The near side person then pulls the rider towards them and, with a straight back and outstretched leg behind, controls the rider as they roll towards the ground. It must be emphasized that the person does not take the weight of the rider, but controls the fall and protects the head. Once the rider is on the ground the horse is carefully led off by the leader and the two team members manage the first aid of the situation.

Emergency dismount example

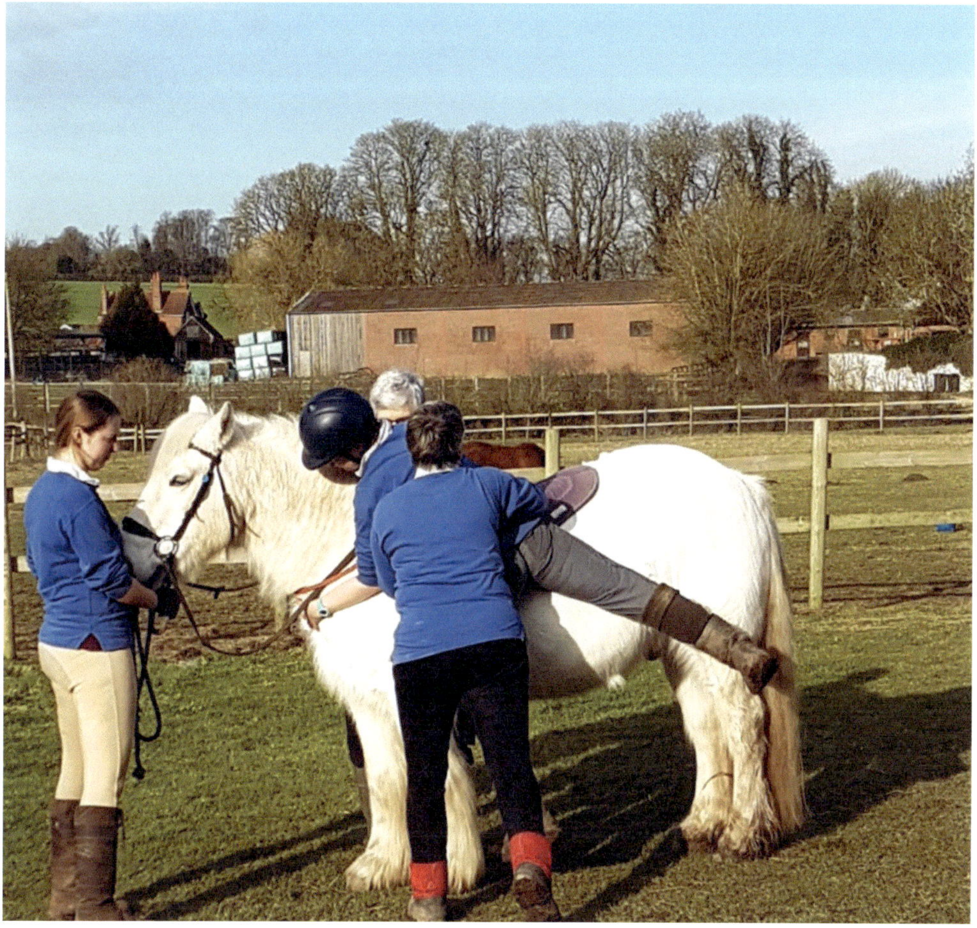

Emergency dismount 5: Controlling the descent

Mark was a 32 year old adult with epilepsy and blindness. Both had been caused by a severe road traffic accident which left him in a coma for several months. He was an inpatient at a local neurological rehabilitation unit. He was attending the centre for physical activity and core strengthening as part of his recovery programme. Whilst riding a large steady cob called Thomas he appeared non responsive to the therapist taking the session. Mark stopped following commands and the therapist moved from the centre of the arena towards him. Mark still wasn't responding and the therapist realised all was not well and called for extra help. The therapist, as the senior on site, kept position at the right leg of the rider and verbally reassured Mark whilst pulling him down to lie on the horse's neck. The fitting started during the lying forwards and the therapist kept Mark safely in this position. The extra help quickly arrived and his feet were removed from the stirrups. The dismount continued but during the roll to the ground the fitting caused the Mark's legs to turn and lie under the horse's belly. Thomas was a little concerned but stood still. Thomas was moved laterally until his back feet were well clear of the prone, fitting Mark and then Thomas was led away. The therapist and assistant managed the rest of the fit and the safe return of Mark to the yard.

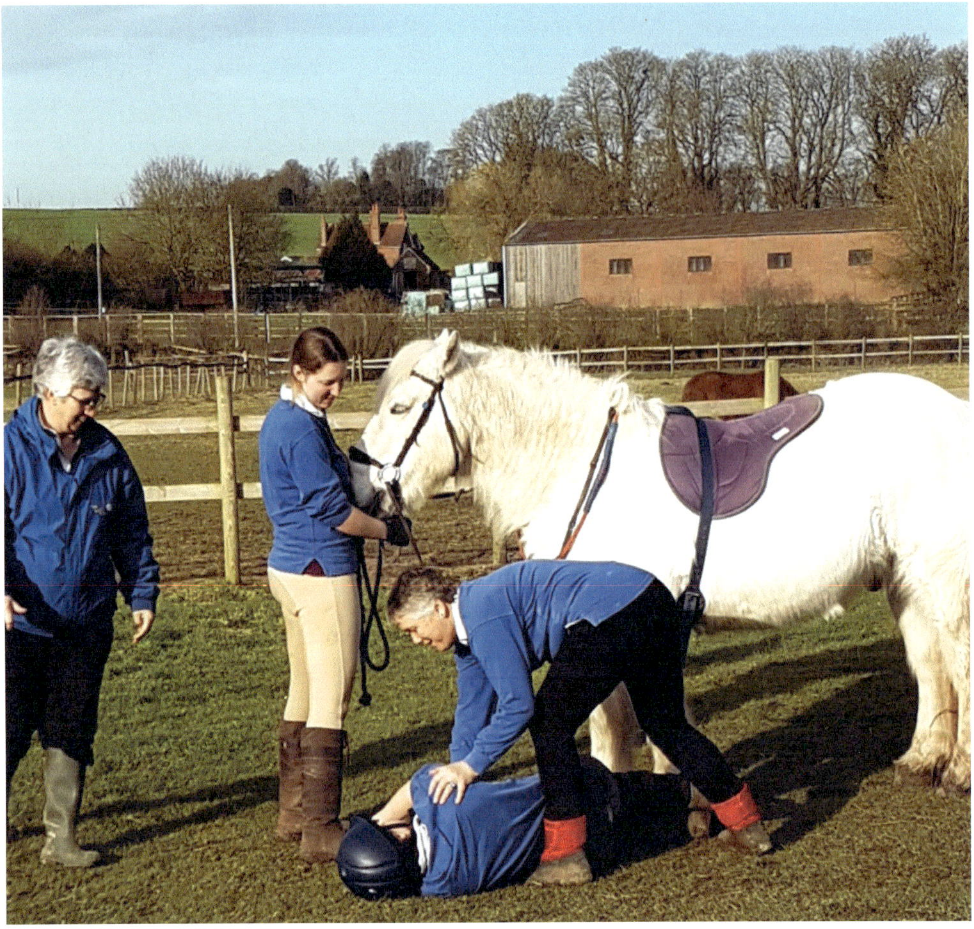

Emergency dismount 6: Safely on the ground

The team, including Thomas, managed well, and Mark soon recovered. He returned to his usual riding sessions and after two months went to live back with his parents in a house with suitable conversions made. He joined a local RDA group and continued his riding.

The team shown in the above pictures all work at a Level 3 centre and emergency dismount training is carried out for all new staff at induction and all staff refresh this annually.

7.4 The organisational umbrella

The umbrella is used in daily living to keep the rain (or sun) off people at a time when they aren't prepared for it in other ways. This is the function of the umbrella here too, but rather than rain it is keeping the provider safe from harm through lack of attention to detail in the daily running of the service.

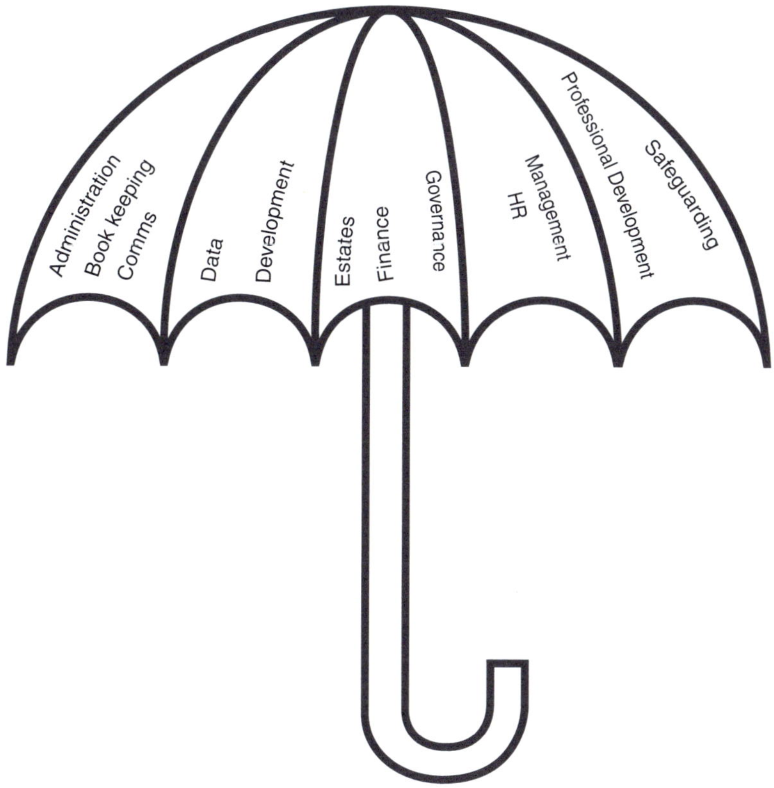

Fig. 24: The Umbrella

The idea of an overarching and protective umbrella of systems is clearly not new for anyone running an approved riding centre, RDA centre, outdoor centre or educational establishment. Regulation and inspection are part of everyday life. This section hopes to bring to light areas that may not yet have been considered over and above normal practice to ensure that everything runs safely.

The umbrella makes reference to the many things required to be an approved provider of outdoor pursuits, riding or health activities and isn't going to surprise those already established. For others considering starting in this field it could be a useful tool for oversight of a service, including the preparation for launching a new provision.

For enquiring funders or potential recipients this offers a checklist against which to measure a potential provision to ensure the whole centre is well managed.

There is an absolute need to have the umbrella in place before planning any sessions. I have developed the one shown in Fig. 24 and have used it over many years and in various settings. It has shown consistency in capturing all areas of importance in charities, public sector organisations and in business.

The explanation of the headings that follows is a list of guidelines that should act as prompts.

7.4.1 Administration

Administration includes all systems which support daily operations. New systems required for this work are those which receive enquiries and applications, inform enquirers, allow timely responses, gather further information prior to assessment, handle information gathered during assessment and support good record keeping. It includes the creation of forms and paperwork needed in addition to those used in the routine provision of the centre. These may include forms for gathering initial information during the enquiry phase and forms for data collection as explained below.

All bookings would be made through such a system of administration to ensure the right facilities, ponies, staff and time are available.

7.4.2 Book keeping and data collection

Clarity about the costs and income generated by this new work will be needed. The book keeping needs to be accurate, reliable and regularly updated. If additional data is to be gathered for consideration by managers, details such as staffing hours or horse hours worked will be recorded. This work would assist in identifying the cost of the provision.

The data being gathered at the start of provision should be reviewed after three months to ensure it is still fit for purpose. Many external agencies deciding whether to refer clients or beneficiaries to a service will expect to see detail about the experience and activity before purchasing, and activity can only be shown through reliable data.

7.4.3 Communication

The new work will need to be advertised in whatever way is considered appropriate. This could be via emails, flyers or posters to local schools or council support officers. The offer from the centre's matrix needs to be clear to those working in the centre so they, in turn, can communicate its content clearly to those outside. Internal communications for any team need to function well, but particularly at times of growth or other change.

Communication also needs to be maintained with external bodies providing supervision or governance in order to keep them informed about progress. Communication with partners and ways of signposting onwards also need to be considered and put in place.

Websites, blogs, Tweets and Facebook posts are all useful but time consuming and, once started, need to be regularly updated.

7.4.4 Development

Keeping development visible encourages the growth of all enterprises. Dreams are good even though not all will be realised. Dreams that are realised, however, show the strength of an organisation to an interested observer. Planning for the future allows organisations to be ready for changes in funding streams whether positive or negative and ensure sustainability. Never underestimate the power of a forward looking plan.

7.4.5 Estates

This refers to the space, range of facilities, horses, other assets and equipment that are available. Its presence on the umbrella list indicates the need to review what can safely be provided using the current level of resource. This should also remind therapy teams to look at the estates with fresh eyes as first impressions matter. What is important to vulnerable people, their families and carers may be different from that which a young person attending for riding lessons will want. Whatever the state of your facilities, remember that a warm welcome will always be paramount in this area of work.

7.4.6 Financial

Whether writing a business plan for a brand new service or considering the financial implications of adding horse based therapy to an existing provision, a financial overview is essential. It should contain an exit strategy and markers to show a sustainable financial position. The type of bookkeeping and budgeting processes required will follow from this financial overview as well as influencing the types of data that will need to be collected.

7.4.7 Governance

The governance required before starting a new therapeutic intervention needs to be commensurate with the level and complexity of the activity provided. Supervision, professional oversight and support for the sessions needs to be appropriate and in place. All professionals will be used to this concept. Anyone hoping to provide in the field of horse based therapy should be encouraged to seek advice on how to arrange supervision in the event that it is required. Risk assessment is an important part of the governance process.

Governance will involve the policies and procedures of an organisation. Workable and useful policies and procedures are an essential tool for all staff at a centre. A statement of the agreed overall way of working and the beliefs held by the organisation are a necessary part of governance for any provision wishing to be taken seriously. Ensuring that policies and procedures are regularly used by all in the team may be a governance challenge for managers.

A policy is an overarching statement about position and outcome and does not need to be wordy or long. A procedure is a step-by-step guide to the actions required in a process.

The umbrella gives a reminder to keep on considering policies and procedures, reviewing regularly and updating periodically to meet changing need. Subjects covered may include: -

- confidentiality
- use of mobile phones during sessions
- safeguarding of vulnerable adults
- facebook contacts
- lone working
- storage of notes made in sessions
- risk assessments
- referring on
- rules on behaviour at the centre
- disclosure of information
- complaints policy and procedure

Teams all hope to provide the perfect session on a regular basis but it must be accepted that often events fall short of this. Preparation for the "slightly less than perfect" session needs a good complaints procedure.

The ability to review and learn through significant events auditing or some similar process is essential to avoid repeating mistakes, improve future working and protect against ongoing or repeated criticisms or complaints.

7.4.8 Human resources

In addition to following normal employment law a new provider may have to consider their approach to volunteers. Qualifications will need to be rigorously checked and the Disclosure and Barring Service (DBS) checks done. The job descriptions or person specifications may need to be reviewed to take the new therapy work into account.

Annual appraisals of staff are seen as good practice within a provision and a centre may be required to show evidence of a working appraisal process before being engaged for provision by a body such as a local authority or school.

7.4.9 Management

Management is always present in the umbrella but only needs to be included here as a reminder not to underestimate the time needed to bring about change.

7.4.10 Professional development

The maintenance of professional knowledge is a growing industry and outside funders will often ask to see the training log of a centre. Many organisations are subject to such scrutiny and centres would be well advised to consider their policy on this. Refresher courses are available in first aid and safeguarding. Log books can be kept and reviewed and lectures attended and recorded.

Lifelong learning for all staff shows that a centre is committed to continuous improvement and many local authorities might be pleased to offer low cost access to training for a centre providing therapeutic intervention to residents of the area.

7.4.11 Safeguarding

Under this heading is an array of areas that need to be safeguarded or are involved in ensuring that safeguarding is being undertaken:-

- staff
- horses
- people attending whether children, adults, vulnerable or learning disabled.
- data
- compliance with Reporting of Injuries, Disease or Dangerous Occurrences Regulations (RIDDOR) and Control of Substances Hazardous to Health regulations (COSHH)
- insurance
- risk assessment

Safeguarding is against theft, lack of confidentiality, damage including by fire or flood, abuse in all its forms and against information technology or cyber crime. Staff need to be trained in confidentiality, safeguarding, risk assessing, moving and handling and management of the fire procedure at the centre.

Records need to be stored in accordance with the Data Protection Act and computer records safely backed up and preferably with a copy held off site. Familiarity with the emergency dismount procedure is a form of safeguarding and should be known and regularly practised by staff.

7.4.12 Partnership working

Partnership working can occur at many levels and may enable activity which isn't possible in isolation. Partnerships will often be important in delivering therapeutic interventions. No matter how good intentions are at the outset tensions may arise if partnership working is entered into without due consideration of differences in approach or expectations.

Such a situation could arise if a centre decided to work with someone to undertake a therapeutic intervention or entered into a partnership with a therapy provider to use a centre's facilities and horses. Agreement would need to be reached about actions such as wearing a hard hat and gloves when working with horses. Some therapeutic interventions require the process to seem natural and providers may consider it safe practice to put a person receiving therapy together with a horse in a round pen with no apparent safety aids in place.

This book is not about making a case for or against the use of hard hats in groundwork, but it is about the consideration of this and the creation of a policy and procedure to which all members of the partnership work. If the approach is to be different in differing settings this needs to be captured in writing.

Lone working may be common practice among riding centres but is not considered safe when managing therapeutic interventions with potentially vulnerable adults and children. Again, there are no hard and fast rules but the advice is that each provider considers their stance on the matter in terms of safety and documents it clearly.

Safe use of social media is a topical area currently and one in which policy and procedure should be met. It may be considered fine for riding coaches to be in contact with their students socially but it would not be considered safe or appropriate in any therapeutic relationship.

It would be more usual to have a "no friends" policy on Facebook for anyone attending any level of intervention. No posts referring to therapy sessions should be allowed however loosely. Even an apparently innocent post such as "it's been a tough day at work" has been considered to breach confidentiality.

Social media activity is best left to the meticulous attention of one careful individual for the organisation. For example, this might be through the management of Facebook and Twitter accounts.

7.5 The "perfect pathway"

The use of the word "perfect" is to encourage the drive towards continual improvement of that which is offered. It will rarely, if ever, be fully achieved. The section that follows is in itself a tool. It provides a checklist covering the preparation, planning and delivery of the pathway in order that nothing is forgotten. The tool can be used by provider, purchaser and participant alike to ensure they are giving or receiving the correct service See fig. 25.

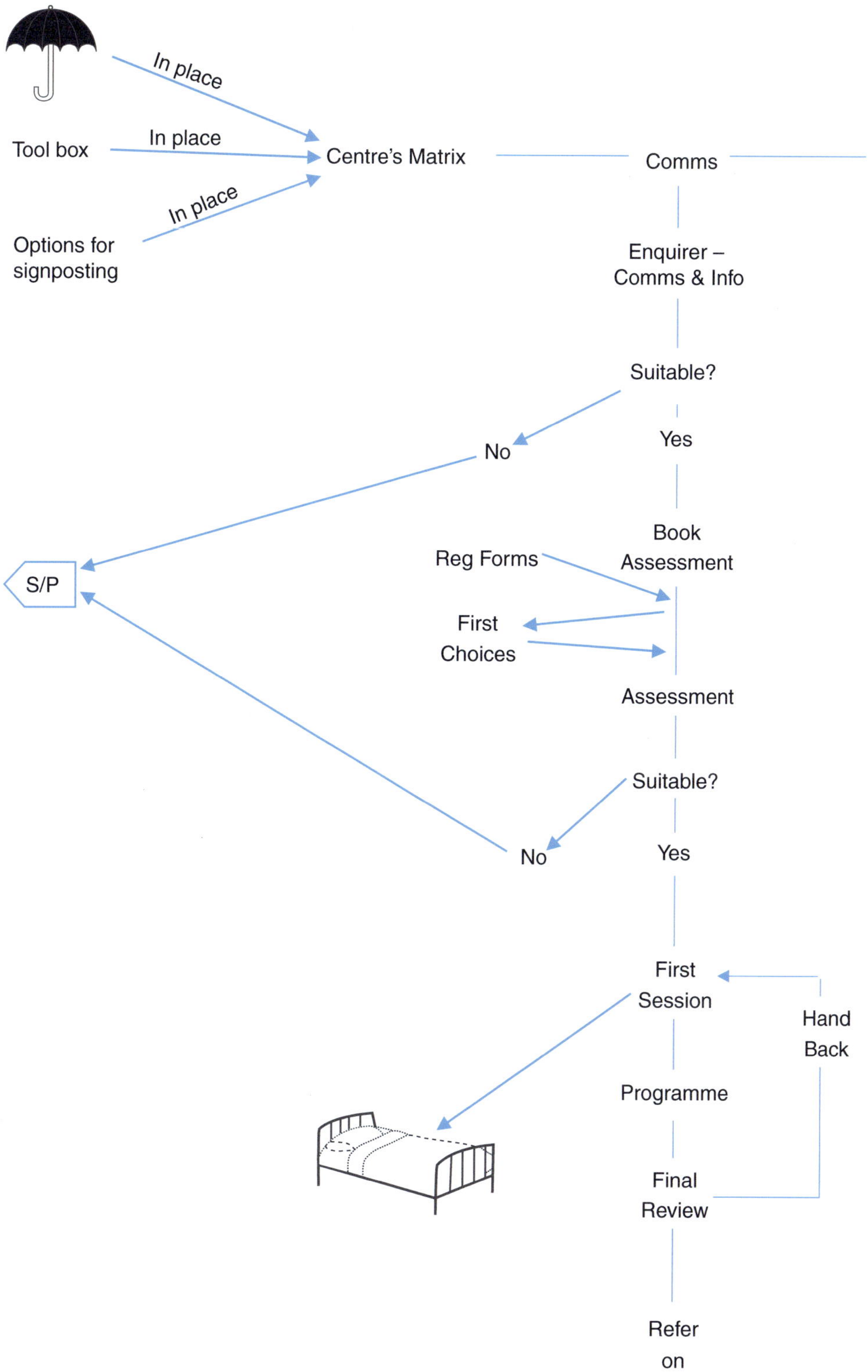

Fig. 25: The pathway of a Perfect Session

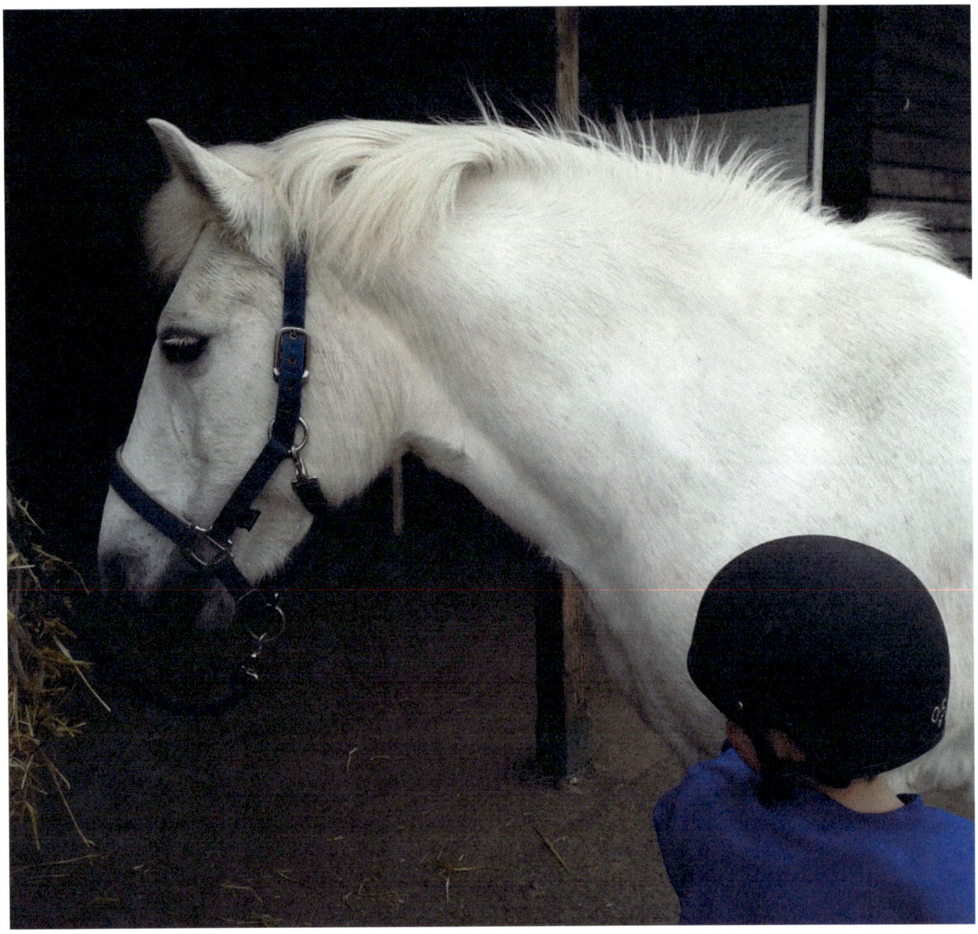

Image 18: The first meeting

To start the pathway the umbrella needs to be confirmed as being in place, the team will be ready and trained and will have some knowledge of what other provisions are available so signposting can happen if needed. The offer matrix will be ready and staff will be aware of how it will work.

7.5.1. The first contact

The first contact with anyone seeking horse based therapy for themselves or for someone else is of great importance. It needs to be professionally managed, non-judgemental and welcoming. Even if the enquiry is not suitable this first contact and the response they receive will colour their impression of horse based therapy as a whole. At this first contact, information is given and gained. The information about the service offered needs to be easily accessible to staff, e.g. through the matrix for the centre, so it can be well communicated to an enquirer. This is also when background information is gained on which later decisions will be made. This will include whether to proceed to an assessment or not. Obviously, if not, this is the first opportunity to use signposting to other services which may be suitable.

7.5.2 The assessment process

The assessment process for a person seeking horse based therapy is a little different from that for mainstream riding. A good assessment requires good choices to have been made beforehand and this requires good information. A registration form completed and returned before the assessment session is invaluable in assisting this process. Once ready, the assessment can be booked with the right person, at the right time, with sufficient time and a suitable horse (including size and temperament), so giving the assessment the best chance of a good outcome.

The purpose of the assessment is:-

- to see whether the centre can offer a therapeutic intervention that will improve the general health and well-being of the individual
- to gain more information to assist in goal setting either then or at a later date
- to see whether the individual understands what is being offered and whether they would like to take it further
- to gain an understanding of what the enquirer hopes therapy will achieve
- to achieve and to confirm that planned outcomes will be realistic
- to decide whether the centre chooses to proceed to work with the enquirer

All therapists should feel free to say no at any point in the process and then do so professionally, either signposting or referring on.

Boundaries for behaviour should be considered at the assessment and this includes not only the person receiving therapy but any person bringing them and family members attending too.

Tensions can arise when the view on what makes a successful outcome is not shared, but this is for the therapist to be aware of and manage through skilful communication.

A warm and professional welcome for the whole party is essential and once all forms are completed the assessment can begin. If the assessment is for a child it is a good idea to leave the parent or carer completing forms and proceed to an activity allowing the child to be observed at a small distance from them.

If there is further information that would be helpful the assessor will decide whether this should be sought at the assessment or at subsequent sessions.

If the person comes with a diagnosis or label an assessor should feel free to review it if it is in their field of expertise and experience. Labels and diagnoses are not always accurate.

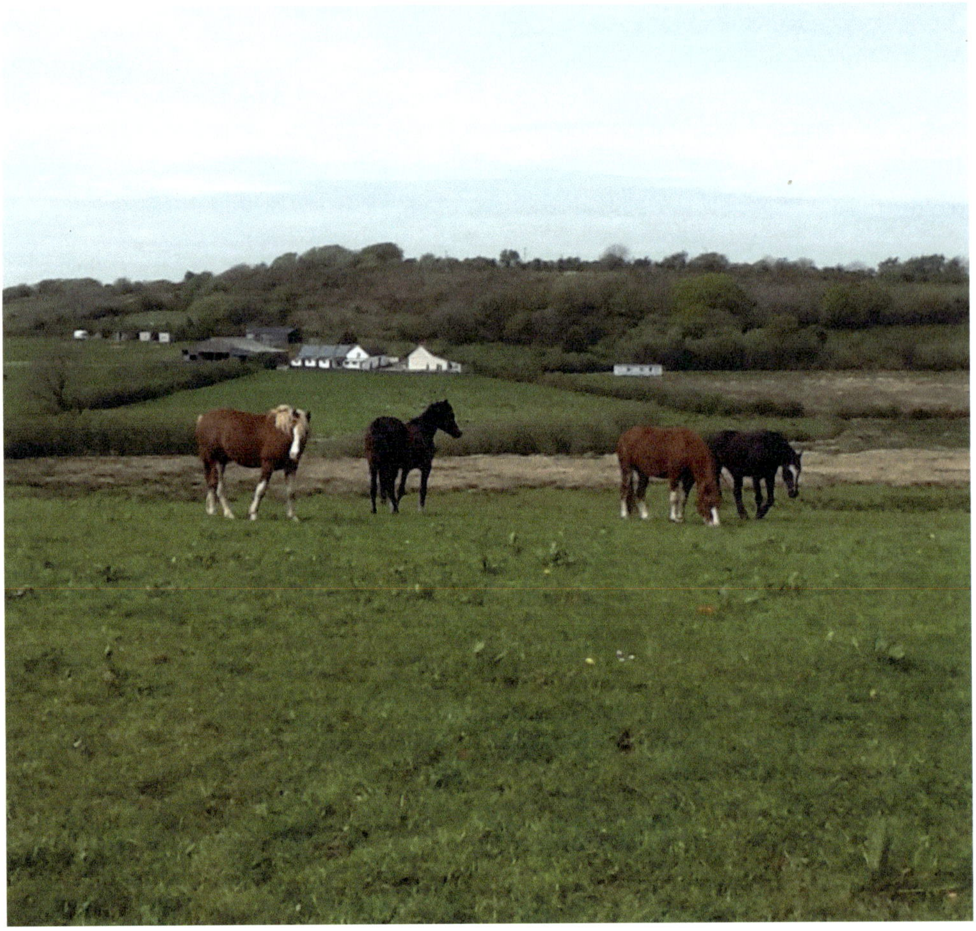

Image 19: Geldings out together after a busy day

At the end of the assessment the assessor should summarise their findings to the individual and other relevant parties, describe what they believe the outcomes could be and the way in which the centre could work with the individual to help that happen. They should also describe what the next steps should be. This may include a discussion about funding options which should be sensitively handled.

If the assessor believes the centre cannot help this individual, they proceed to signposting or referring on.

If the decision is made to proceed the person can be booked in for a suitable, regular slot and activities chosen that interest both the individual and therapist.

Using the matrix of the centre during the assessment is a very useful way of ensuring good consideration of the options available. Once ticks are placed in the boxes this matrix becomes part of the notes of the person in therapy and, after photocopying, could be given to them to remind them on what the programme outline will be based.

7.5.3 The first session

The information gained, and agreement reached at the assessment, enables the preparation for the first session to be made. The therapist, and possibly the therapy assistant who will be taking the sessions, can decide on which tools to use, which horse and which activity or mix of activities will be best. The outcomes can be considered ready for discussion and confirmation at the first session.

The first session is an opportunity to build relationship, test an approach which can be changed if needed, and confirm the programme in terms of length and goals, preferably with completion of a recovery star. The first session may be deemed a success simply if the person attends. It does not need to be complex. Long journeys all start with small steps.

7.5.4 Putting each session to bed

At the end of each session there are certain considerations and actions required. The horse needs to be allowed to recover whether this has been a particularly emotional session or not. This is best achieved by turning out for "herd time" as described in Chapter 5.

Notes need to be written and placed in safe storage and staff need to process what has happened and whether it went well or not. A cup of tea in the office with other team members is a good way of unwinding. Supervision should be in place for more awkward sessions even if it is only on an occasional or as needed basis.

7.5.5 The programme and its review

Recording what happens in sessions is essential. It allows progress towards goals to be recorded. In the event of the progress slowing or stopping it also allows re-evaluation to take place, once again giving the opportunity to reset to a different programme or to refer on. Reviewing progress towards goals can seem intrusive and time consuming but without it there can be no reliable review.

Review can also be a way for families to come to terms with their situation, perhaps surprising them with good news or sometimes helping them to understand what is really going on with their family member.

The programme offered should always have an end point identified e.g. "during this term" or "until they can".

A final review should be undertaken, preferably one week before the end of the actual programme. All success needs to be recognised and applauded. The reason for taking the final review before the end is that it allows consideration of the decision that then needs to be made, i.e. whether to carry on with or to finish therapy, to engage with another programme, or to refer on to a different provider for a different aspect or level of horse based therapy.

The pathway as shown above can, of course, be localised for any centre using it. It should be easily available to all staff and volunteers together with the completed offer matrix for the centre.

7.6 In summary

Whilst the therapy involved in Horses and Human Health is complex it is hoped this book will help to explain why this is so. It is further hoped that the reader will understand how they

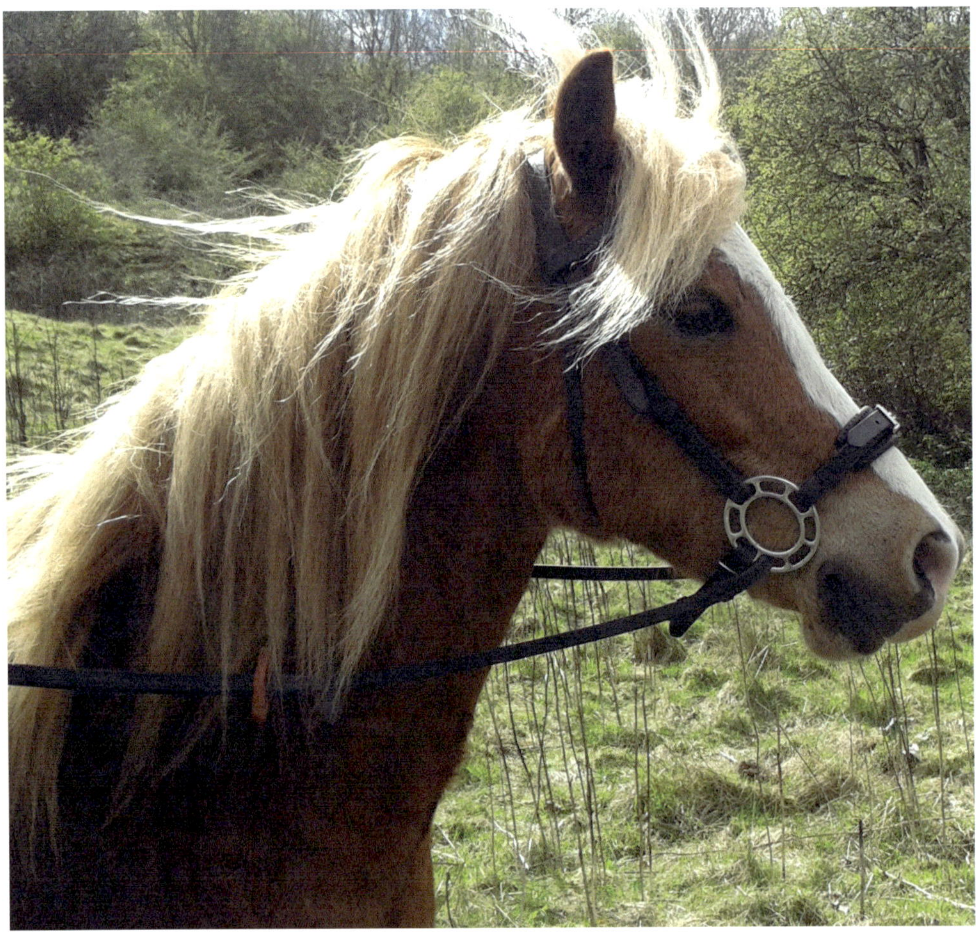

Image 20: Welsh Section A, Raci Crackerjack, in his bitless bridle and ready for a session on a spring day

could be part of the provision of this powerful therapy and want to be involved. More therapy provision means this highly effective intervention is made available to more people, more data is created for review and more lives improved as a result.

Without the 25 years clinical and equine experience on which this book has been based, I would still be seeking ways of helping people beyond that which medicine can offer.

Case study 7

The office was rung by a very distressed mother who was sobbing. Her son, Simon, had been excluded from his Special Educational Needs School some two weeks previously and no placement had been found for him. Simon was a 12 year old with epilepsy, a known autistic spectrum condition and worsening behaviour as he grew tall enough to bully others.

The charity has access to bursaries for young people in need and it was decided to go straight ahead with offering an assessment for temporary placement using the bursary initially. The intention was to seek the Special Education Needs placement funding once Simon was safe again.

Simon came to the yard three days later. He was smiling the minute he came up the drive and was looking at the ponies. Mother was surprised. Simon's behaviour throughout the assessment was entirely appropriate, as is so often the case. His high functioning autism was not displayed, his behaviour was within the normal range. It was noted that there was little eye contact but he was happy to groom, poo pick and then ride. This latter was done with a back pad only on this occasion.

During the assessment the scale and size of the land available to the Charity was shown to Simon and a short walk led into the area of woodland on the site. Simon liked all the countryside signs, was excited at seeing a squirrel and found fox poo fascinating. He liked the site of the hide which is an outdoor classroom and thought he would be interested in learning some countryside skills as well as learning to work with horses.

Made in the USA
Monee, IL
12 September 2026

63115051R00079